AF522639

# EMERGING ENVIRONMENTAL CONTAMINANTS AND GLOBAL HEALTHCARE SYSTEMS

# EMERGING ENVIRONMENTAL CONTAMINANTS AND GLOBAL HEALTHCARE SYSTEMS

*Editors*

**Prof. (Dr.) Shyam Narain Pandey**
*Professor*
*Department of Botany*
*University of Lucknow*
*Lucknow (U.P.) (India)*

**Murtaza Abid**
*M.Sc. (Botany), M. Phil.*
*GATE (Life Sciences)*
*CSIR-NET/JRF (Life Sciences)*
*ARS-ICAR/NET (Plant Physiology)*
*JRF-CSIR*
*Department of Botany*
*Lucknow University, Lucknow, (U.P.)*
*(India)*

**Prof. (Dr.) Syed Rais Haider**
*Professor and Head*
*Department of Botany*
*Shia P.G., College*
*Associated with Lucknow University*
*Lucknow (U.P.)*
*(India)*

**Dr. Sabiha Kazmi**
*Associate Professor*
*Department of Botany*
*Shia P.G. College, Lucknow*
*(U.P.) (India)*

**Dr. Mohd. Zahid Rizvi**
*Senior Assistant Professor*
*Department of Botany*
*Shia Post Graduate College, Lucknow*
*(U.P.) (India)*

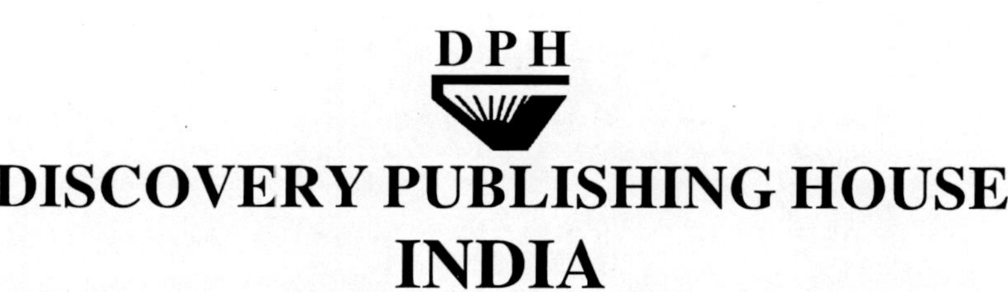

**DISCOVERY PUBLISHING HOUSE**
**INDIA**

*Published by:*

**DISCOVERY PUBLISHING HOUSE**
4383/4B, Ansari Road, Darya Ganj
New Delhi-110 002 (India)
*Phone* : +91-11-23279245; 23253475; 43596065
*E-mail* : discoverybooksindia@gmail.com
discoverypublishinghouse@gmail.com
namitwasan9@gmail.com
*web* : www.discoverypublishinggroup.com

*First Edition:* **2023**

**ISBN: 978-81-959169-2-4**

**Emerging Environmental Contaminants and Global Healthcare Systems**



*Printed at:*
Infinity Imaging Systems
Delhi

## Dedication

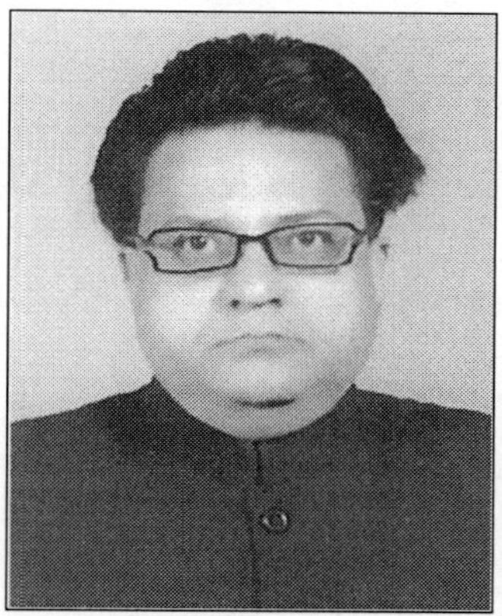

**This book is dedicated to my beloved parents**
**Professor (Dr.) M.M. Abid Ali Khan (Father)**
**and**
**Dr. Aziz Abidi (Mother)**

Murtaza Abid
Editor

# Preface

"Emerging Environmental Contaminants and Global Healthcare Systems" cover all aspects of emerging contaminants in the environment which threaten life on Earth. Further emerging contaminant remediation in a pressing need due to the ever increasing pollutants in the environment, and it gained a lot of scientific and public attention due to its high effectiveness and sustainability. The discussions of the book on the bioremediation of these contaminants are covered from the perspective of proven technologies.

The delicate balance exists between environmental quality and quality of life, both human and animals are important for healthy existence and sustenance of life on Earth. In the recent past, chemical compounds ubiquitous in the environment, have received considerable attention. These include personal care products, pharmaceutical compounds, micro-plastics, perfluoroalkyl substances, nanoparticles and others. Collectively, they have come to be known as 'chemicals of emerging concern' (CEC) or emergent contaminants (EC). The revelation of their occurrence in the environment has been made possible by the continuing development of robust analytical tools for detection and quantification. Though their transport and fate may not be completely understood, toxicity studies have shown these emergent contaminants to be toxic even at very low concentrations. These reports have sparked debate over the occurrence of these chemicals in the environment and the implications on global health. Several technologies have been proposed in the recent years to sequester emerging contaminants from environment. This book explores these issues and the chapters have been organized in a logical sequence. The first three chapters describe the impact of soil contamination on human health, a review on emerging contaminants and environmental and health impacts on air pollution. Chapter 4-8, the reader is furnished with Biotic, abiotic and ecological factors of river, the impact of environmental toxins on cardiovascular system, effect of environmental factors and climate change on Mycobacterium tuberculosis, environmental toxicants: types, sources and effects, green nanotechnology and environment. Chapter 9-14 deal with the Ocean Biome: Diverse Habitats and Marine Life, Microbes in the Environment, Ocean Acidification and its Impacts, Conception of Sustainable Development, Conception of Urban Ecology, Contaminants in the Environment: Water Pollution, whereas chapter 15-18 evaluate Ecology and Environmental Contaminants: Challenges and Way Forward, Food Contamination: An Overview, Environmental Contaminants: Review, Bioremediation as an Expedient Biotechnological Strategy for the Mitigation of Phenolics.

Suggestions that can improve the future editions of this book are highly welcome. We hope you enjoy the reading of this book.

**Editors**

# Acknowledgements

First, I would like to thank all the contributors and reviewers of this book who were part of this project and observed it emergence from concept to reality. Your support through reading, writing, reviewing and proof reading is acknowledged. I appreciate my family's unwavering support of my pursuits as much as it takes away valuable time that would have been spent together. It is from the interactions with my mother Dr. (Mrs.) Aziz Abidi, Ex-Senior Assistant Professor of Botany, Shia P.G. College, Lucknow, India and my father Professor (Dr.) M.M. Abid Ali Khan, Department of Botany, Shia P.G. College, Lucknow, India that inspired my interest in this subject. Their inspiration is recognized by all editors of this book. I appreciate your persistent interest and readiness to step in at any point of this book. Last but not least, I thank the Almighty Allah and His last Apostle for His providence throughout the course of this project in the form of book.

Thank you all.

**Murtaza Abid**
**(*Editor*)**

# Contents

Pages: 1-9
**Emerging Environmental Contaminants and Global Healthcare Systems**
*Editors:* **Prof. (Dr.) Shyam Narain Pandey; Murtaza Abid**
**Prof. (Dr.) Syed Rais Haider; Dr. Sabiha Kazmi; Dr. Mohd. Zahid Rizvi**
*ISBN:* **978-81-959169-2-4**
*Edition:* **2023**
*Published by:* **Discovery Publishing House, New Delhi (India)**

# Impact of Soil Contamination on Human Health

**Karneshwar Gholia, Mrityunjay Mishra**
**Lovy Singh Bist and Amit Gupta**

## ABSTRACT

*Soil is one of the most important components on this planet, whose necessity is comparable to that of air itself. All the life has evolved from the nurturing of soil. Over the years man has been found guilty for the overexploitation of soil to satisfy his greed. This has led to the pollution of soil which has turned into a major concern and which cannot be neglected for how important soil is. This chapter covers the causes behind the pollution of soil and the negative impacts that soil pollution poses on human health.*

***Keywords:*** *Soil, Necessity, Pollution, Human and Health.*

## INTRODUCTION

Soil is called the fragile skin of the earth, it the uppermost layer that is abundant with vital nutrients and minerals. It is a non-homogenous mixture containing a variety of substances, which gives the soil its typical nature. It is a mixture containing mud, slit, clay, humus, small pebbles, minerals, organic matter and even living organisms, these are the factors that provide dynamism to the soil. The composition and properties of soil is continuously changing because the different components in soil are active and react chemically [1].

Soil is one of the most important features of our ecosystem as most of the food we consume directly or indirectly comes from soil. Plants require

**Department of Biotechnology, Graphic Era (Deemed to be) University, Dehradun-248001 (India)**

minerals and water for their growth which they obtain from soil. It is also a home for various animals and microorganisms. Higher beings are dependent on these plants that grow from soil, which transport the minerals obtained from soil at the time of consumption. Hence, the importance of soil is to be greatly emphasized. The formation of soil is a very slow process involving thousands of years in the making. Weathering is the process known for the formation of soil. It the process of breaking down of rocks into finer particles and then accumulation of these particles over an area, different from the place of origin through the action of wind, water and gravity. Weathering can be physical, chemical or biological [2, 3].

- **Physical weathering** involves the mechanical method that includes any changes in the temperature, frost or abrasions.
- **Chemical weathering** occurs when the minerals in the rock react with the atmospheric air or water over a period of time, which leads to a change in their chemical makeup causing their breakdown.
- **Biological weathering** is the process of breakdown of rocks by the activity of any living being, such as plant roots or burrowing animals.

There are different factors that affect the process of soil formation as they are related to the process of weathering. Some of these include: temperature, topography, climate, and the quality of the parent material (rocks).

## SOIL POLLUTION

The composition of soil is what makes it nurturing and provides its ability to generate life. Substances mix with the soil can bring about changes in the chemical composition of the soil, which may lead to the degradation in the quality of the soil. This is known as soil pollution, and the substances that mix with the soil and change its chemical composition and texture are called soil pollutants. These pollutants are also responsible for reducing the productivity of fertile soil thus hampering the process of sustaining life. These can be radioactive substances, toxic compounds, insecticides, pesticides, solid organic matter, etc. All the unprocessed waste that is dumped into the soil will cause pollution to a massive amount and threaten the life of humans, animals and other living beings that depend upon the soil one way or the other, also toxic pollutants in soil like lead, mercury and other chemicals causes the widespread of diseases like leukaemia, cancer, neuromuscular blockages, depression, etc. [4-6].

Hence, soil pollution is a very big challenge for our environment today. It has therefore become very important to continuously monitor over the quality of soil and prevent its contamination from any sort of polluting substance. Also, serious efforts should be made to carry out the conservation of soil through activities like, planting of tress, avoiding overgrazing, regulation of crops, etc. [7-9]

## Types and Sources of Soil Pollution [10-12]

Soil is a non-renewable natural resource, which humans have been continuously overexploiting to satisfy their needs. Land areas have been used as a contamination sink since the very beginning of the industrial revolution. Chemicals and minerals occur naturally in the soil to an extent, but if their amounts exceed the recommended levels, health of humans, plants and animals will be compromised it can detrimental as soil pollution is directly related to the loss of biodiversity. Soil pollution can be categorized into two types:

- **Specific pollution:** the area to be accounted for pollution is comparably smaller with particular causes which are easily identifiable. Polluted areas around cities, old factory sites, around roadways, illegal dumps, sewage treatment plants, can be categorized under specific pollution.
- **Widespread pollution:** these include pollution over a large-scale area, the cause behind which are difficult to be identified. These involve the spreading of pollutants through air-ground-water system, which are also responsible to affect the human health and environment.

The sources and causes of soil pollution should be realized in order to preserve the fertility and productivity of soil [10-14]. Some sources that are responsible for polluting soil are mentioned below:

(a) **Waste from industries:** industrial activities produce a large amount of waste. These include many toxic chemicals, carcinogens and heavy metals. When the waste from these industries is directly dumped into the nearby areas, all the toxins from these waste mix with the soil and bring about change in the natural soil composition. Industrial waste includes heavy metals like Pb, As, Cd, Hg-all of these are responsible for causing severe diseases like leukaemia and cancer.

(b) **Dumping of e-waste and medical waste:** both e-waste, flammable retardants, and infectious waste discarded as biomedical waste contain toxins that directly mix with the soil and are absorbed by the plants growing in the contaminated area, they eventually enter our ecosystem, contaminating the food chain.

(c) **Landfills:** leachate that is generated by the decomposition of waste is the most important source of pollution in landfills. It penetrates into the soil and brings about change in the natural composition of soil. The negative impacts of landfills remain even years after the landfill has been closed.

(d) **Indiscriminate use of fertilizers and pesticides:** when chemical products like fertilizers and pesticides are unconsciously sprayed over the farming area, they invariably change the composition of soil by the overaccumulation of certain minerals and metals into the soil. They also contain other toxic substances. The plants growing in the contaminated soil take up these chemicals and when they are consumed, they cause diseases. When these chemicals mix with the groundwater, they also cause water pollution.

Except for these, mining, deforestation, dumping of domestic waste, discard of untreated sewage, is other causes behind soil pollution.

## CASE STUDY - 1

**Relation between heavy metal soil pollution and stomach cancer – a Case Study in Hangzhou City, China:**

Stomach cancer is also known as gastric cancer and can affect any part of the stomach. Mostly the stomach cancers (about 90-95 %) are said to be adenocarcinomas. It is a severe burden and nearly half of the world's cases are reported in China.

The increase in the exposure of heavy metals along with other radioactive elements in the soil has been noticed since the beginning of industrialization. A reported study based on the diagnosed cases of stomach cancer in Hangzhou city in with the quantitative characterization of geographical areas in association with their associativity to the heavy metals, was carried out in 2018. The result showed that: Cadmium (cd) is one of the severe pollutants in the soil along with others like lead (Pb). In the city of Hangzhou higher, cases were reported in the central city, which was the area exposed to a greater content of these heavy metals. Lesser cases were reported in northeast and southwest areas. The ratio of suffering males and females was found to be (2.2:1).

It was concluded that though the associativity of stomach cancer in association with cadmium was not significantly noted but it is very clear that heavy metals have significant impacts on stomach cancer risks.

### Impact on Humans Health

Soil pollution is a major concern as it affects the life of plants animals and humans. Crops and plants that are cultivated in contaminated soil absorb the toxins present in the environment which causes damage to the food and habitat of all living organisms. Soil pollution is also harmful for health of human beings. These effects are sometimes visible for a shorter period, but they may also become grave and stay longer.

- **Short term effects:** Direct exposure to soil contaminants can lead to skin diseases such as skin allergy or irritation, pimples and acne and some common problems such as headache, nausea, vomiting, difficulty in breathing, pain in the chest, wheezing etc. These are known as the short-term effects of soil pollution.

- **Long term effects:** In some cases, it may lead to harmful conditions such as skin cancer in which red patches appear on the skin which might bleed, some contaminants present in soil increase the risk of leukaemia which is mainly caused by chemicals like benzene. Other contaminants present in soil can also lead to serious issues like kidney damage and liver problems. These serious and harmful conditions caused by the contaminants are also termed as long-term effects of soil pollution.

**Harmful Effects of Heavy Metals [15, 16]**

Heavy metals discharged in the form of industrial waste are dumped in the soil which get seeped inside and sometimes mix with ground water. This contaminated water when used for drinking purposes leads to various health hazards. Similarly, the crops grown in such kind of affected soil also results in health deterioration. The effects of some heavy metals are discussed as under:

- **Cadmium:** Cadmium (Cd) is a naturally occurring metal. It usually exists in the environment in its mineral form which is combined with other elements like oxygen, chlorine, or sulphur. Cadmium is a heavy metal and is generally disposed of in landfills, open burning, dumping in the form of metal waste which is hazardous in nature. When a person breathes in high level of cadmium from air or eats food and drinks water having high amount of cadmium results in cadmium poisoning. Exposure to cadmium for a short period of time can cause curable problems such as fever and muscle pain and exposure for a longer period result in problems like kidney failure and bone diseases.
- **Lead:** Lead (Pb) is found in nature in ores with other metals. Exposures to lead can cause problems such as anaemia, weakness, kidney and brain damage and longer exposures to lead can even lead to death. Pregnant women who are exposed to lead also expose their foetus which results in damage of the nervous system of the baby. Exposures to lead for a longer period of time can also result in lead poisoning, also known as plumbism and saturnism which can cause memory problems, abdominal pain, constipation, infertility.
- **Arsenic:** Arsenic (As) naturally occurs in soil and is present in atmosphere in the form of airborne dust. Effects of long-term exposure to inorganic Arsenic can be seen in the form of chronic arsenic poisoning, skin lesions and skin cancer and is also related with cardiovascular diseases and diabetes. The immediate effects of acute arsenic poising include vomiting, abdominal pain, diarrhoea, blood in the urine, stomach pain, numbness, muscle cramping and death in extreme cases.

As, Arsenic is the natural component of the Earth's crust, it is widely distributed throughout the environment in the air, water and land. This Arsenic, present in the soil/land, get mixed with the ground water and pollute the soil as well as the ground water. People get exposed to the inorganic form of this highly toxic metal by drinking contaminated water, using contaminated water in food preparation and irrigation of food crops, industrial processes, eating contaminated food and smoking tobacco. It should be noted that contaminated groundwater is also a threat to public health. Many countries of the world like Argentina, Bangladesh, Chile, China, India, Mexico and the United States of America are having high levels of inorganic Arsenic in the ground water. Fish, shellfish, meat, poultry, dairy products and cereals can also be the dietary sources of arsenic. Tobacco smokers can also be exposed to the natural inorganic arsenic content of tobacco as tobacco plants take up arsenic naturally present in the soil.

## CASE STUDY - 2

### Dietary survey conducted in Nanning (October, 2002)

Presence of Cadmium (Cd) and Lead (Pb) in soil is responsible for the damage of nervous system especially in children. Studies have shown that the food chain is the main pathway of Cadmium and Lead transfer from the environment to humans. This fact was exposed in a dietary survey conducted in Nanning in October 2002. The main objective of the survey was to measure Cd, Fe, Cu, Zn, Ca and Pb along with the urinary indicators of renal dysfunction Albumin (ALB), N-acetyl-beta-D-glycosaminidase (NAG), Beta-2-microglobulin and Retinol-binding protein in the samples of soils, plants(vegetables), urine and blood of humans. The results of the study showed that the local residents living in the area where soil was contaminated with metal mixtures suffered with renal dysfunction, and the dose response curve was a bit altered by the mixed contamination of Cd and Pb as well as the intake of other minerals.

## CASE STUDY - 3

### Assessment of heavy metal pollution on human health – a Case Study around an industrial zone in Neyshabur, Iran

Potential human health risks are noted due to heavy metal pollutants of soils in the industrialization area, which is therefore a matter of attention. Research in attempt to realize and monitor the status of heavy metals such as arsenic (As), cadmium (Cd), lead (Pb), chromium (Cr), nickel (Ni), along with other distinct pollutants, was conducted. The use of various indices like pollution index (Ipoll), contamination factor (CF) and geo-accumulation index (Igeo), was made.

The procedure for carrying out this investigation included the sample soil collection from 60 soil surfaces from four different areas namely, (north, south, east and west), in the Khayyam industrialization zone. The soil samples were mined from depths of 10-20 centimetres.

According to the results it was noted that the concentration of heavy metals ranges in (mg/kg), with the observations- 8.84, 1.9, 37.66, 15.77 and 57.33 for As, Cd, Cr, Ni and Pb respectively. The concentrations of these heavy metals- As, Cr, Ni and Pb with exception of Cd were reportedly high in the southern area where the industrial zones were more active. Lesser concentrations of the cadmium metal (Cd) were noted in the north, east and western regions. According to the indices of geo-accumulation (Igeo), contamination factor (CF) and pollution index (Ipoll) the concentration of the heavy metals was observed in the following order: Cd> As> Pb> Ni> Zn.

It has hence been proven that industrial activities in the Khayyam industrialization zone have shown an elevated effect on the concentration of metals in the soil, hence polluting it. Therefore, it is important to monitor the soil around the areas including and surrounding the industrialization zones, especially for Cd and As metals, to reduce potential risks to human health and environment.

**Controlling Measures**

Soil pollution is an emerging problem that requires urgent attention. We need to take appropriate measures like adopting the policy of 3R's: Reduce, Reuse, and Recycle, and many more, to tackle this serious problem as all of the living ecosystem could be at stake, since, soil is the most importing thing in this world, because it's serves as a habitat to a lot of organisms and also, we grow our vegetables in/on soil. We also need to protect the soil quality because all plant and trees grown on soil, and they release oxygen for us to breathe. As the quality of soil is getting worst day-by-day, due to all this pollution, it's getting difficult for plant to grow in polluted soil and also, it's getting difficult for many organisms to live and depend on this soil.

Some measures that will help us to control and treat the soil pollution are listed below:

- **Adopting the 3R's policy:**

  The 3R's policy is a very good initiative. We should Reduce, Reuse and Recycle everything. This will help to reduce the solid waste and also by reusing and recycling, a lot of minerals can be saved as there's no need to create more quantity of items that can be recycled and reused. Also, this will lead to less waste from manufacturing plants.

- **Microbial treatment of soil:**
  We can use microbes present in soil naturally, by isolating and culturing them in lab, and adding them to the polluted soil. These microbes will remove all the harmful pollutants from the soil.
- **Not using pesticides:**
  Farmers should reduce the use of pesticides. Pesticides damage the nutritional value of the soil and also add harmful toxins to the soil, which makes it unfit for farming and kill many good microorganisms and insects, present in the soil.
- **Stop using chemical fertilizers:**
  Farmers should stop the use of chemical fertilizers, instead should use Bio-Fertilizers. Chemical fertilizers cause a lot of soil pollution. Bio-Fertilizers and manure should be used, as it not only helps in crop cultivation, it also increases the fertility of soil and its nutritional value.
- **Afforestation:**
  Planting more trees will protect the soil from landslides and soil erosions.
- **Crop Rotation & Mixed Cropping:**
  These techniques help in increasing the fertility of soil.
- **Proper disposal of waste form Factories:**
  Solid waste from factories should not be dumped directly into wasteland. Waste should be treated properly before being disposed. It should be filtered and only biodegradable material should be disposed in waste dumps.
- **Domestic waste management:**
  People throw their domestic waste in open, empty plots, and sometime on roads, all of this causes a lot of soil pollution. People should dispose their domestic waste properly, for example, they should throw the waste in dumpsters, or in government trucks that come every day to collect the waste from houses. We should also reuse material like plastic bags, bottles and glassware. We should not throw the non-biodegradable items in open, as they take time or mostly can't be broken down by the microorganisms naturally and hence, causes a lot of soil pollution. Rather, we should throw such items in dumpster, provided by government everywhere, specifically for plastic items only, so that they can be recycled.

## REFERENCES

1. Pepper, I.L. The Soil Health: Human Health Nexus. Critical Reviews in Environmental Science and Technology 2013; 43: 2617-2652.

2. Oliver, M.A. and Gregory, P.J. Soil, Food Security and Human Health: A Review. European Journal of Soil Science 2015; 66: 257-276.
3. Brevik, E.C. Soils and Human Health: An Overview. In: Brevik EC, Burgess LC, Editors. Soils and Human Health. CRC Press; Boca Raton, FL, USA: 2013, 29-56.
4. Buck, B.J., Londono, S.C., McLaurin, B.T., Metcalf, R., Mouri, H., Selinus, O. and Shelembe, R. The Emerging Field of Medical Geology in Brief: Some Examples. Environmental Earth Sciences 2016; 75: 449.
5. Brevik, E.C., Pereg, L., Steffan, J.J. and Burgess, L.C. Soil Ecosystem Services and Human Health. Curr Opin Environ Sci Health. 2018; 5: 87-92.
6. Brevik, E.C. and Sauer, T.J. The Past, Present, and Future of Soils and Human Health Studies. Soil. 2015; 1: 35-46.
7. Baumgardner, D.J. Soil-related Bacterial and Fungal Infections. J Am Board Fam Med. 2012; 25: 734-744.
8. Pelser, C., Dazzi, C., Graubard, B.I., Lauria, C., Vitale, F. and Goedert, J.J. Risk of Classic Kaposi Sarcoma with Residential Exposure to Volcanic and related Soils in Sicily. Ann Epidemiol. 2009; 19: 597-601.
9. Krishna, A.K. and Mohan, A.R. Distribution, Correlation, Ecological and Health Risk Assessment of Heavy Metal Contamination in Surface Soils around an Industrial Area, Hyderabad, India. Environ Earth Sci 2016; 75: 411.
10. Certini, G., Scalenghe, R. and Woods, W.I. The Impact of Warfare on the Soil Environment. Earth Sci Rev 2013; 127: 1-15.
11. Li, C., Zhou, K., Qin, W., *et al.* A Review on Heavy Metals Contamination in Soil: Effects, Sources, and Remediation Techniques. Soil Sediment Contam 2019; 28: 380-394.
12. Wei, B. and Yang, L. A Review of Heavy Metal Contaminations in Urban Soils, Urban Road Dusts and Agricultural Soils from China. Microchem J 2010; 94: 99-107.
13. Song, Q. and Li, J. A review on Human Health Consequences of Metals Exposure to e-waste in China. Environ Pollut 2015; 196: 450-461.
14. Egwa, A.G., Ferdinand, P.U., Nwalo, F.N. and Unachukwu, M.N. Mechanism and Health effects of Heavy Metal Toxicity in Humans. In: Karcioglu, O, Arslan, B, eds. Poisoning in the Modern World. London: Intech Open 2019: 1-23.
15. Kim, K.W., Kabir, E. and Jahan, S. Exposure to Pesticides and the Associated Human Health Effects. Sci Total Environ 2017; 575: 525-535.
16. Steffan, J.J., Brevik, E.C., Burgess, L.C. and Cerdà, A. The Effect of Soil on Human Health: An Overview. Eur J Soil Sci 2018; 69: 159-171.

**Corresponding author: Dr Amit Gupta, Associate Professor, Department of Biotechnology, Graphic Era (Deemed to be) University, Dehradun, India.**
**Email id: dr.amitgupta.bt@geu.ac.in**

Pages: 10-14

Emerging Environmental Contaminants and Global Healthcare Systems

*Editors:* Prof. (Dr.) Shyam Narain Pandey; Murtaza Abid

Prof. (Dr.) Syed Rais Haider; Dr. Sabiha Kazmi; Dr. Mohd. Zahid Rizvi

*ISBN:* 978-81-959169-2-4

*Edition:* 2023

*Published by:* Discovery Publishing House, New Delhi (India)

# Emerging Contaminants *Review*

**Bharat Rohilla, Rakesh Pant, *Nirmal Patrick and Amit Gupta**

## ABSTRACT

*The substances present in small quantities in Environmental matrices that causes adverse health effect on the matrices life due to prolonged exposure could be named as Emerging Contaminants. This article summarize the data from several reports and researches done while efficiently explaining the causes, effects, methods of screening, methods of removal, their effects on the Antimicrobial resistivity phenomenon. While researchers struggled to develop new methods and enhancing the traditional ones for effective screening and removal techniques, the rise in concentration was dramatic due to increase in the usage of the products responsible for their ultimate source due to industrialization. The screening concludes some commonly used techniques for suspect/specific molecules and for non-target screening for a wider range detection.*

***Keywords:*** *Environment, Health, Contaminants and Screening.*

## INTRODUCTION

The organic and inorganic matter present in water bodies that discern harm to environment and human health can be regarded as Emerging Contaminants. Increase in usage of chemical substances in modern world on global scale, like disinfectants, additives, nano materials, hospital waste, hazardous non-biodegradable material due to rapid industrialization and

Department of Biotechnology, Graphic Era (Deemed to be) University, Dehradun-248001 (India)

*Department of Quality, Eureka Forbes Ltd. Lal Tappar, Dehradun-248140 (India)

urbanisation leads to eutrophication of the chemicals in water medias. The medication used by the general mass is also flushed out from body and later on joins the rivers and lakes. Compounds like Perfluorinated compounds, Disinfection byproducts, Gasoline Additives, Manufactured Nano materials, Human and Veterinary Pharmaceuticals and Sunscreen/ Ultraviolet filters are the chemicals which constitutes the- Emerging Contaminants.

These contaminants are harmful and toxic in certain levels to human health and environment. For instance, PFCs can be potentially but sparsely carcinogenic. Many reports also states the association between the serum level of PFCs and reproductive dysfunction in general population, including breast feeding, infertility and semen quality in humans. Reports based from DNBC program suggests that exposure to PFOS and POAS may lead to a decline in reduction of fecundity in the general mass. Disinfection byproducts like THMs also may have carcinogenic effects resulting in colorectal and bladder tumour, along with suspection of risk factors for infertility, fetal loss, long gestational duration and poor fetal growth and fetal anomalies. DBP exposure may also negatively influence normal sperm concentration and morphology but motility percentage is retained. Gasoline additives like MTBE can be rapidly absorbed by inhalation, exposure with thermal absorption and ingestion of contaminated water may also lead to exposure to these additives. Studies shows that MTBE is a suspected carcinogen, exhibits a potential toxicity on human body leading to testicular, uterine, and kidney cancer and also harm kidney, immune system, liver and central nervous system.

Materials at nano scale produced having the approximately size of 1-100 nm also takes up part in consistency for Emerging Contaminants. [1] Silicon dioxide, carbon nanotubes are some examples, mostly present in products like sunscreen, agricultural chemicals, healthcare materials and many more. However, even pharmaceuticals drugs with no nano particles ends up being as contaminants. In the present time, animals and human's usage of drugs has increased dramatically. Since most drugs leave the body by excretion and ultimately ends in water sources. Both veterinary and human pharmaceutical drugs end up as encouraging the contaminants. Further, these drugs effect aquatic life, may be harmful even for humans later on due to fishes and marine life as one of staple food in many countries. While talking about drugs, non-pharmaceuticals like hygiene and personal care products including skin and hair care contains sunscreens and ultraviolet filter chemicals, both in cosmetic and non-cosmetic products. They ends up in water by daily needful chores of mass like bathing, washing clothes etc. and studies have shown their connection with endocrine disrupting system in marine life.

**Screening methods for Emerging Contaminants**

Emerging contaminants being in smaller quantities makes them quite difficult for screening and identification in samples, requiring higher levels of sensitivity and resolutions for probes and sensors. Due to growth in research in technological fields, the progression in sensitivity and resolution in mass spectrometers in recent years provides the possibility to detect a broad range of organic compounds in a single procedure [2]. While suspect screening gives much more details regarding specific contaminating matter, non-target screening provides details on wider range of chemicals. Sample preparation is usually first and critical step before the analysation as it may greatly affect the factors for truer aspects in terms of results. Some common used techniques could be solvent extraction and solid phase extraction for liquid samples.

The traditional techniques were used to analyze very small fractions of substances requiring selectivity and had major complicated matrices. They had limiting factories like restriction of detection of non-selected samples even if present in more concentration. One of recent discoveries, High Resolution mass spectrometers (HRMS) allowed detection of all identifiable substances i.e. a broader range of substances were correctly identified correctly. Use of some HRMS techniques like Quadrupole Time of Flight (QToF) and Orbit-trap mass spectrometers, when couples with chromatographic techniques (gas/liquid) promoted identification of unknown contaminating chemicals [2].

After screening, removals of contaminants are usually done by water and waste water treatment processes, membrane treatments [3]. While studies suggests that evidence is not enough to state casual associations between emerging contaminants and adverse effects on human body, some experiments performed on animals concludes long-term chronic exposure is seldom and the adverse effects must not be ignored [1].

Water samples are usually are more analysed in the all of environmental matrices for both selective/suspect and non-target screening of contaminants and unregulated chemicals. SPE technique is generally the preferable method for extraction of water samples due to its high capacity and ability to remove complex interferences with various solid phase sorbents, Oasis HLB technique being specific[3]. Oasis WAX, HR-X and C-18 are the other available sorbents which commercially could be used for extraction of compounds from water samples. A combination of sorbents while SPE can be helpful to extract compounds at a far greater range. However even these sorbents come with some limiting factors, for instance, Oasis HLB SPE was found somewhat less effective with log Dow chemical's due to HLB being less effective for polar interactions occurring via hydrogen-bond and dipole interaction, Graphitized carbon SPE was found suitable for extraction of Organochlorine pesticides (OCP's), herbicides and phthalates but not very effective for elation of analytes from sorbents.

To reduce the loss of chemicals while extraction, for water samples a direct injection without any sample preparation was suggested, which while tested after a filtration technique was able to identify some new contaminants which were previously not considered as contaminants. Sample extraction from air, sediment and sludge uses different types of techniques like microwave extraction, ultrasonic solvent extraction, ultra sonication with DCM etc.

**Antimicrobial Resistance due to Emerging Contaminants**

Living organisms are well known for adapting, increasing resistance to unfavorable factors to support life, due to the phenomenon known as "Evolution". Microbes, both pathogenic and non-pathogenic develop resistance to their growth inhibiting stimulus and chemicals, leading to arise in difficulties for treatments. AMR raised rapidly in the past century due to inappropriate use of antibiotics in both, human and veterinary sector [4]. This lead to two contributing factors in the already wide field of Emerging contaminants as *Antimicrobial resistance* and *Emerging organic contaminants*, the antibiotics used are passed through body and excreted through urination, which then reaches the streams and on one side increase the concentration of organic contaminants, while also encourages AMR as more and more microbes start growing under the influence of these antibiotics.

As the microbes gets more resistant to the already existing antibiotics, it severely decreases the number of options of treatment available for patients infected against the same microbes, thus need for new version of antibiotics to be effective for the mutated micro-organism.

Most common sources of these contaminants are Hospital waste, Household waste from people using these antibiotics, Wastewater treatment plant, Agriculture and aquaculture, Industrial waste, urban runoffs; these sources mostly dumps the waste in water streams which leads to AMR and EOC.

**Removing Contaminants- Methods**

As the more and more studies suggested the rising concern of emerging of contaminants, and their adverse effects on human health due to chemicals such as endocrine disrupting compounds (EDC's) and pharmaceuticals (PhACs)/personal care products (PPCPs) etc., certain steps were needed to screen and effectively remove the concerned substances. Failure in removal of these problematic contaminants may cause damage to nervous system, liver and kidneys on prolonged exposures, according to reports, along with cancer risks. Different types of contaminants may need additional or special steps because of not able to get removed by waste water treatment processes. Not only that but inorganic contaminants or EOCs, likes of Cr(VI), As(V) and perchlorate(ClO4-) are getting more common in drinking water and causing water quality and health issues[3].

Many reports incline in the failure of completely reomovage of CECs by conventional WTPs and WWTPs.

## CONCLUSION

Since the large variety and wider ranges of Emerging contaminants present in ever Environmental Matrices, and the concern of effects on human health, animal health and marine life, researchers rapidly began to develop methods for screening and the purpose of removing. Source of Emerging contaminants varies according to the type of substance but some common can be named as waste from municipal and households, along with industrial and hospital waste.

## REFERENCES

1. Overview of Emerging Contaminants and Associated Human Health Effects by Meng Lei, Lun Zhang, Jianjun Lei, Liang Zong, Jiahui Li, Zheng Wu, and Zheng Wang Department of Hepatobiliary Surgery, First Affiliated Hospital of Medical College, Xi'an Jiaotong University, Xi'an, Shaanxi 710061, China.
2. Sample Preparation Techniques for Suspect and Non-target Screening of Emerging Contaminants Parvaneh Hajeb, Linyan Zhu, Rossana Bossi, Katrin Vorkamp, Aarhus University, Department of Environmental Science, Roskilde, Denmark.
3. Removal of Contaminants of Emerging Concern by FO, RO, and UF Membranes in Water and Wastewater Jiyong Heo1, Sewoon Kim2, Namguk Her1, Chang Min Park3, Miao Yu4, Yeomin Yoon.
4. The Role of Emerging Organic Contaminants in the Development of Antimicrobial Resistance Izzie Alderton a, *, Barry R. Palmer b, Jack A. Heinemann c, Isabelle Pattis a, Louise Weaver a, Maria J. Gutierrez-Gines a, Jacqui Horswell b, 1, Louis A. Tremblay d, e.
5. Photo Enhanced Degradation of Contaminants of Emerging Concern in Waste Water Olalekan C. Olatunde a, b, Alex T. Kuvarega c, Damian C. Onwudiwe a, b.
6. Review Marine Microplastic Debris: An Emerging Issue for Food Security, Food Safety T and Human Health Luís Gabriel Antão Barbozaa, b, c, N, A. Dick Vethaakd, e, Beatriz R.B.O. Lavorantea, b, Anne-Katrine Lundebyef, Lúcia Guilherminoa, b.
7. Survey of 218 Organic Contaminants in Groundwater Derived from the World's Largest Untreated Wastewater Irrigation System: Mezquital Valley, Mexico Luis E. Lesser a, b, 1, Abrahan Mora c, *, 1, Cristina Moreau c, Jürgen Mahlknecht c, Arturo Hernandez-Antonio b, Aldo I. Ramírez c, Hector Barrios-Pin~a c.
8. Emerging Contaminants in Urban Groundwater Sources in Africa J.P.R. Sorensen a,*, D.J. Lapworth a, D.C.W. Nkhuwa b, M.E. Stuart a, D.C. Gooddy a, R.A. Bell a, M. Chirwa b, J. Kabika b, M. Liemisa c, M. Chibesa c, S. Pedley D.

**Corresponding author: Dr Amit Gupta, Associate Professor, Department of Biotechnology, Graphic Era (Deemed to be) University, Dehradun, India.**
**Email id: dr.amitgupta.bt@geu.ac.in**

Pages: 15-23
**Emerging Environmental Contaminants and Global Healthcare Systems**
*Editors:* **Prof. (Dr.) Shyam Narain Pandey; Murtaza Abid**
**Prof. (Dr.) Syed Rais Haider; Dr. Sabiha Kazmi; Dr. Mohd. Zahid Rizvi**
*ISBN:* **978-81-959169-2-4**
*Edition:* **2023**
*Published by:* **Discovery Publishing House, New Delhi (India)**

# Environmental and Health Impacts of Air Pollution

**Mrityunjay Mishra, Lovy Singh Bist**
**Karneshwar Gholia, Amit Gupta**

## ABSTRACT

*There are activities that violate the original nature of the ecosystem causing many unwanted changes in the environment leading to many lifestyle problems as well. One such major concern over the past few years has been the increase in the level of pollutants in the atmospheric air causing air pollution. Air pollution is a serious issue which demands our attention because pollutants present in the air are leading to crisis like global warming. Pollutants can harm us when present in high concentration, causing serious health and environmental issues. This book chapter presents a comprehensive account of air pollution, emphasizing on the impacts of polluted air on our health and environment.*

***Keywords:*** *Ecosystem, Environment, Health, Air and Pollution.*

## INTRODUCTION

Air is what we breathe in and out. It is one of the five basic elements of nature, which is colorless, tasteless and cannot be seen, unlike the other states of matter and can only be felt. Air is a mixture of different gasses present in our atmosphere. Different gasses are present in a specific amount/ concentration which constitutes our atmosphere and this makes our earth the only planet to support life. Nitrogen is the most abundantly present gas with 78.04% concentration, oxygen is 20.94%, 0.93% argon, 0.04% carbon dioxide and various other gasses present in small traces. Also, air contains variable amount of water vapor. The air around us is a blanket, supporting

**Department of Biotechnology, Graphic Era (Deemed to be) University, Dehradun, (India)**

life promoting activities that cater the need of all living beings and plays a vital role to promote all biotic and abiotic factors. Humans and animals require air to breathe; plants consume the carbon dioxide during photosynthesis to prepare their food. The dissolved air in water bodies provides life to the aquatic beings. The dynamics of air regulates the climate of an area. All such factors make air an undisputable factor for the sustainability of life on earth [1, 2].

Due to the unsuppressing urge of mankind for making their lives easier with the help of advancement in science, has had many significant and negative impacts over the years. This has eventually led to the degradation in the quality of our environment and health, the basic reason behind which is pollution. As there are a certain percentage of different gasses precent in the atmosphere, any change in this composition leads to a variety of problems. Air pollution is the referred to as any sort of physical, chemical or biological change in the air. When the quality of air is dampened by pollution, we can observe many immediate and long-term consequences. The most scaring factor about air pollution is that, one may not suspect the presence of pollutants in the air cause simply no one can see air. Although air pollution is quite visible sometimes when one may notice dense smog lingering over a city. Smog is the mixture of smoke consisting of particulate matter mixed with the fog. This smog is considered to be quite dangerous as it reduces the visibility level causing many miss-happenings [3, 4].

## SOUCRCES OF AIR POLLUTION

As the presence of particulate matter in air cannot be marked, hence it becomes necessary to identify the various sources behind air pollution. There are two major types of air pollutants which are classified as [5, 6]:

- **Primary Pollutants:** these are the particles that are directly emitted by the identifiable sources of pollution such as automobiles, industries, burning of fuels and natural activities like volcanic eruptions and storms. These are present in both gaseous and particle. The particulate matter can be of various sizes or physical state depending upon its physical state, mainly – aerosol, dust, mist, smoke, fume and fly ash. There are five basic types of primary pollutants that majorly contribute in the pollution of air, they are:
  - Oxides of carbon ($CO_2$, CO)
  - Oxides of Sulphur ($SO_2$)
  - Oxides of nitrogen ($NO_2$, $NO_3$, NO)
  - Suspended particulate matter (SPM)
  - Hydrocarbons
- **Secondary Pollutants:** when the primary pollutants are released in the atmosphere, they start to react chemically with the other pollutants,

resulting in the formation of secondary pollutants. Hence the primary pollutants give rise to the secondary pollutants. Some of these are – nitric acid, sulphuric acid, formaldehydes, carbonic acid, ozone, peroxy-acyl-nitrate (PAN), etc.

Some major sources of air pollution [7, 8] are listed as follows:

**The burning of fossil fuels:** We require to burn fossil fuels such as coal, petroleum, gasoline, etc. to produce energy required in household, generation of electricity and transportation. The burning of these fossil fuels releases carbon monoxide in huge amounts along with other toxic pollutants. These pollutants are very dangerous as they cause respiratory and cardiac diseases. It is noticed that most of the air pollution is caused by the burning of these fuels.

**Wildfires and Burning of Agricultural waste:** The changing climatic factors and thunderbolts are responsible for the forest fires. These wildfires cause the increase in level of PM.25 in the air along with harmful gasses and pollen creating smog. Other than these the burning of farm residues and agricultural practices like slash and burn method of farming also leads to air pollution. The spraying of fertilizers and pesticides also aids in polluting air as some of these gets mixed with the air and cause numerous health related issues.

**Use of chemical and synthetic products in households:** Air inside our homes, schools or offices can be more polluted as outside. The household products we use contain volatile organic compounds. (VOCs) which are very harmful and pollute the air. Also, inadequate ventilation, uneven temperature, and smoking of tobacco, room heaters etc. also pollute the air inside.

**Industrial Emissions:** Industries most commonly use wood and coal as their primary energy source for the production of their goods. This leads to the emission of innumerable amount of particulate matter along with gasses like nitrogen dioxide, Sulphur dioxide, carbon monoxide, etc. which degrade the air quality more than we can imagine. These pollutants released from the industries cause irritation in eyes and throat and even chronic illness.

**Automobiles:** Using of vehicles for transportation, especially in urban cities is a major cause behind air pollution. The fuel that is used in automobiles release various gasses such as carbon monoxide and nitrogen dioxide along with hydrocarbons and particulate matter consisting of CFCs (chlorofluorocarbons). These pollutants emitted from automobiles are very dangerous and they are held responsible for the creating holes in the ozone layer also causing global warming.

### Microbial Decaying Process

Industries and manufacturing hubs directly discard their waste products in the surrounding areas. These contain a lot of organic matter which are acted upon by microorganisms such as bacteria and fungi, as a result of their microbial activity they release many toxic gasses like ammonia, methane, Sulphur dioxide, which not only produce bad odor and contaminate the surroundings but inhalation of these toxic gasses can be fatal. Some other factors that cause air pollution include- burning of domestic waste, construction and demolition, volcanic eruptions, etc. these causes of air pollution has left everyone thinking and worried about their health as the increasing rate of air pollution has made breathing of fresh air next to impossible. Thus, people should take this very seriously and initiate methods to prevent any sort of pollution- taking immediate measures has become an absolute necessity.

## IMPACT OF AIR POLLUTION ON HUMAN HEALTH

As we know, Air pollution is caused when air gets contaminated by any physical/chemical/biological agent. So, as we breathe, these agents are also sucked into our body and they cause a lot of damage. Every year, millions of deaths are reported due to air pollution, which makes it the biggest environmental health risk. Most vulnerable people are the children, elderly people and people with existing health issues. Children have a very weak immune system as it is in developing stage. Due to this, they are very sensitive towards air pollution. Breathing polluted air for long period of time can cause severe damage to their respiratory system and can cause diseases that could stick for a long time or even for the entire lifespan. In elderly people, due to ageing, their immune system also becomes weak and hence they also become very vulnerable towards the air pollution. They are also more sensitive as they may already have some diseases which can increase the damage caused by air pollution.

There are two types of health effect of air pollution [9-11]:

- **Short term Effects:** Short exposures to air pollution can lead to temporary problems such as irritation in eyes, skin infections, inflammation in nose and throat, wheezing, coughing, difficulty in breathing, headache, dizziness and nausea. If not taken care properly, these problems can lead to some serious risks.
- **Long term Effects:** Exposure to air pollution for a longer period of time can cause serious problems such as asthma, pneumonia, bronchitis, lungs and heart related problems and may leads to cancer. Long term effects are chronic and last for years or lifetime and can be fatal.

Example: On Diwali, every year, people burn fire crackers which alone cause around 30% of the entire year's air pollution. It raises the Air Quality

Index so significantly that, for many days, many cities have to be completely locked down. Air around these days is so polluted that people can't even breathe without mask. It causes irritation and redness in eyes, suffocation, cough, headache, short term lung diseases and even asthma in some people. It also causes education loss as school also have to remain shut for some time, since air quality index is so high that it's super dangerous for students' health.

## CASE SUDY - 1

**Air pollution and human health in Kolkata -** Urban and metropolitan cities have continuously faced the setbacks of air pollution and Kolkata being a megacity has had no exception to this. An annual average of air pollutants including- RPM, SPM, $NO_2$ and $SO_2$ were made by performing the Exceedance Factor method (EF) to check the ambident air quality, which clearly was not much remarkable due to the presence of these pollutants. There are total 17 ambient air qualities monitoring stations in Kolkata out of which 15 fall under the critical category, whereas the remaining 12 locations fall under the high concentration category polluted by high nitrogen-dioxide concentrations. 4 locations record high concentrations of RPM, 13 come under the basic pollutant category. The cause behind this high level of pollutants were identified which and it was observed that automobiles (51.4%) and industrial sources (24.5%) have been the major source for degrading the air quality; these also include the dust particles (21.1%).

To recognize the adverse effect of these pollutants, a health assessment was also conducted, with a detailed questionnaire prepared for the local dispensaries which fall under the critical areas of the air ambident pollution level. The survey was made in 3 dispensaries with 100 participants giving their feedback and was noted that respiratory diseases (85.1%) has surpassed waterborne diseases (14.9%). Which include respiratory infections (ARI-60%), chronic obstructive pulmonary disease (COPD-7.8%), upper track respiratory infection (UTRI-1.2%), acid fast bacillus (AFB-3.4%) and influenza (12.7%).

Thus, these are some alarming rates of air pollution and it has become the need of the hour to continuously monitor over the quality of air by regular checks and following measures to control the pollution of air.

## EFFECTS OF AIR POLLUTION ON ENVIRONMENT

Besides affecting the human health, air pollution can also cause a variety of environmental effects [12-14].

- **Acid rain-** there are many pollutants present in the atmosphere, these pollutants harm the environment in various ways. One such hazardous result is acid rain.

  Acid rain is a term which means the deposition of a mixture of acidic components present in air with rain, which leads to the increment in the number of hydrogen ions which causes lowering down of pH.

General pH of acid rain ranges from 4.0 to 5.0. Acid rain occurs due to the discharge of Sulphur dioxide and nitrogen oxide, which reacts with the water molecule present in the atmosphere and produce acids. These toxic acidic gases come from vehicles and factories in form of smoke. Acid rain has been shown to have unfavorable impacts on forests, freshwater and soil by killing microbes, insects and aquatic life forms. It is also responsible for the weathering of rocks. When acidic rainwater falls on rocks such as marble, limestone or chalk, it causes breaking down of minerals and changes its chemical composition.

Acid rain is also a major problem for monuments. When the sulphuric acid and nitric acid present in the rainwater, comes in contact with material such as marble, limestone etc., the calcite present in them starts to dissolve which leads to the removal of material and makes the surface rough. In some studies, it has been clearly observed that the great monuments like Taj Mahal have been affected due to acid rain. The suspended particulate matter, released in the smoke from the Mathura oil refinery discolors the Taj Mahal's white marble, making it yellow. In other words, acid rain corrodes the marbles and this phenomenon stated as "marble cancer".

- **Crop and forest damage-** Air pollution can damage crops and trees in a variety of ways. Ozone gas present at the ground level damages crop by entering in leaves during normal gas exchange process. It causes yellowing of leaves, cell injury, and tiny spots of bronze or dark red color. This directly affects the growth and cultivation of agricultural crops and commercial forest yields. Pollutants present in air also affect the soil by changing the pH due to which toxic salts off elements like aluminum mix with the soil and makes it barren.
- **Effects on wildlife-** Air pollution are harmful for humans and also a major concern for wildlife. It can cause serious problems search as lung damage, heart diseases, inflammation and cancer. Studies have shown that for birds with long term exposure to pollution, there was reduced egg production and hatching and the babies that were born have small body size and organelle dysfunction. Besides this, gases such as ozone damages plants and trees that birds rely on for food and shelter.
- **Depletion of ozone layer-** Sun is the major source of heat energy on earth. It produces sunlight which contains ultraviolet radiation which is harmful in nature. Direct exposure to ultraviolet rays can lead to problems like wrinkled skin which is also known as early aging of skin. Ultraviolet rays can also cause eye problems as their exposure to eyes can lead to burning of cornea. These ultraviolet rays get absorbed

by a shield like layer present in the atmosphere known as ozone layer. It is a region on earth's stratosphere that absorbs most of the Sun's ultraviolet radiation (About 97 to 99 percent of UV rays). Due to the release of chemical from industries, the ozone layer was being depleted continuously, which leads to the direct exposure off harmful UV radiation in the environment from the depleted spots present in the ozone layer also known as ozone hole. These holes In the ozone layer are caused by some air pollutants such as chlorofluorocarbon (CFCs), hydrochlorofluorocarbon (HCFCs) and halons.

For example; the chemical used in refrigerants, coolants like chlorofluorocarbon contain chlorine atoms. When these chemicals are released in the atmosphere, the chlorine present in it destroys the ozone layer. A single atom of chlorine can destroy thousands of ozone molecule and the increasing level of ultraviolet radiation in the atmosphere can also lead to skin cancer.

- **Global climate change-** Due to the increase in population, the requirements of people have also been increased. More people mean more demand for fuels and essential sources. As a result, industrialization has expanded which has led to massive cutting down of trees and exploitation of natural resources. Consequently, there is an increase of gases like carbon dioxide, methane, water vapors etc., also known as greenhouse gases. The sun rays enter the atmosphere of the earth and warm the planet's surface. The gases present in the atmosphere absorb the radiation and prevents it to return to the space and the heat gets trapped in the atmosphere of the earth which results in warming up of the planet. This phenomenon is termed as Greenhouse effect. The greenhouse gases are emitted from human activities such as burning fossil fuels for generation electricity and heat, increase in transportation, extensive use of fertilizers for agriculture, use of refrigerants etc., resulting in the increase in the average temperature of the world which is also known as Global Warming.

## CASE STUDY - 2

### Impacts of Modifiable factors on Ambident Air Pollution – A Case Study of Covid-19 Shutdowns

The adversity of the spread of the deadly virus- COVID-19, offered a novel opportunity to carry out and measure the levels of modifiable factors on the ambident air pollution in real time. The data was obtained through Real-Time Affordable Multi-Pollutant sensor packages which were acquired through Pittsburgh and Pennsylvania. Data was also obtained through Environmental Protection agency regulatory monitors. Based on the usage of land the RAMP locations were divided into four site group. Then the concentration of the pollutants such as PM2.5, CO and $NO_2$, were made in comparison to the regular business days before the era of the epidemic and the shutdown.

It was observed that as the traffic level on the roads had significantly decreased and also industries and factories were shut down, so a significant decrease in the concentration were observed and the result was quite surprising. The PM concentration significantly had fallen down by 50%, though there were not many changes observed in the concentrations of CO and PM2.5B in the industry related area.

**Measures to Reduce Air Pollution-** In today's time, there is an urgent need to reduce air pollution as, day by day, it is causing more and more damage to humans, animals and environment. It is possible to bring Air Quality Index significantly low by simply implementing small changes in our lifestyle. Some of these changes are:

- **Using public transport more often:**

  Vehicle causes a lot of air pollution. The more are the cars on road, the more will be air pollution caused by them. To reduce this, we should use public transport like buses, train, autos, etc., instead of driving our own car. This help's in reducing the number of vehicles on road and hence, less air pollution.

- **No Deforestation:**

  Trees help in reducing air pollution as the take the carbon dioxide form the air and release clean oxygen in the environment. Therefore, we should not cut down trees and focus on planting more and more trees.

- **Less usage of harmful chemicals:**

  Goods manufacturers should not use hazardous chemicals, as they release harmful gases in air, which, if inhaled, causes severe damage to humans, animals and even damage plants.

- **Don't burn firecrackers:**

  People burn a lot of firecrackers on Diwali and even in marriages, and smokes from these firecrackers causes a lot of air pollution. This smoke gets mixed up with the fog and creates "smog", which is very harmful as it makes breathing very difficult and also reduces the visibility. So, people should understand the health risk caused by these firecrackers and should stop using these.

- **Reduce smoking:**

  When a person smoke's a cigarette, they release a lot of smoke which is very harmful for the environment, as it causes air pollution. Also, Smoking is very harmful as it leads to a lot of respiratory diseases. So, smoking is not good for person doing it and also for the people in the surrounding's.

- **Farmers should not burn remains of the crop after harvesting.**
- **Stopping forest fires.**
- **Using filter on chimney.**

## REFERENCES


1. Ahmed, H.W. and Alamire, J.H. A review of Machine Learning models in the Air Quality Research. Int J Adv Res Comput Eng Technol 2020; 9 (3): 30-36.
2. Althuwaynee, O.F., Balgoun, A.L. and Al Madhoun, W. Air Pollution Hazard Assessment using decision Tree Algorithms and Bivariate Probability Cluster Polar Function: Evaluating Inter-correlation Clusters of PM10 and other Air Pollutants. GI Sci Remote Sens 2020; 57 (2): 207-218.
3. Athira, V., Geetha, P., Vinayakumar, R., Soman, K. Deep Air Net: Applying Recurrent Networks for Air Quality Predict. Procedia Comput Sci 2018; 132: 1394-1403.
4. Ayturan, Y.A., Ayturan, Z.C. and Altun, H.O. Air Pollution modeling with Deep Learning: A Review. Int J Environ Pollut Environ Model 2018; 1 (3): 58-62.
5. Zheng, M., Salmon, L.G., Schauer, J.J., Zeng, L., Kiang, C.S., Zhang, Y., *et al.* Seasonal trends in PM2.5 source Contributions in Beijing, China. Atmos Environ. 2005; 39(22): 3967-76.
6. Kurokawa, J., Ohara, T., Morikawa, T., Hanayama, S., Greet, J.M., Fukui, T., *et al.* Emissions of Air Pollutants and Greenhouse Gases over Asian Regions during 2000-2008: Regional Emission Inventory in ASia (REAS) Version 2. Atmos Chem Phys Discuss. 2013; 13(4): 10049-123.
7. Oderbolz, D.C., Aksoyoglu, S., Keller, J., Barmpadimos, I., Steinbrecher, R., Skjøth, C.A., *et al.* A Comprehensive Emission Inventory of Biogenic Volatile Organic Compounds in Europe: Improved Seasonality and Land-cover. Atmos Chem Phys. 2013; 13(4): 1689-712.
8. Shen, H., Huang, Y., Wang, R., Zhu, D., Li, W., Shen, G., *et al.* Global Atmospheric Emissions of Polycyclic Aromatic Hydrocarbons from 1960 to 2008 and Future Predictions. Environ Sci Technol. 2013; 47(12): 6415-24.
9. Veras, M.M., Caldini, E.G., Dolhnikoff, M. and Saldiva, P.H. Air Pollution and effects on Reproductive-system Functions Globally with particular Emphasis on the Brazilian Population. J Toxicol Environ Health B Crit Rev. 2010; 13: 1-15.
10. Cairncross, E.K., John, J. and Zunckel, M. A Novel Air Pollution index based on the Relative Risk of Daily Mortality associated with short-term Exposure to Common Air Pollutants. Atmos Environ 2007; 41: 8442-54.
11. Shahrabi, N.S., Pourezzat, A., Ahmad, F.B., Mafimoradi, S. and Poursafa, P. Pathologic Analysis of Control Plans for Air Pollution Management in Tehran Metropolis: A Qualitative Study. Int J Prev Med 2013; 4:995-1003.
12. Molina, M.J. and Molina, L.T. Megacities and Atmospheric Pollution. J Air Waste Manag Assoc 2004; 54: 644-80.
13. Chen, B. and Kan, H. Air Pollution and Population Health: A Global Challenge. Environ Health Prev Med 2008; 13: 94-101.
14. Brucker, N., Charão, M.F., Moro, A.M., Ferrari, P., Bubols, G., Sauer, E., *et al.* Atherosclerotic Process in Taxi Drivers Occupationally exposed to Air Pollution and Co-morbidities. Environ Res. 2014; 131: 31-8.


---

**Corresponding author: Dr Amit Gupta, Associate Professor, Department of Biotechnology, Graphic Era (Deemed to be) University, Dehradun, India.**
**Email id: dr.amitgupta.bt@geu.ac.in**

Pages: 24-33
**Emerging Environmental Contaminants and Global Healthcare Systems**
*Editors:* **Prof. (Dr.) Shyam Narain Pandey; Murtaza Abid**
**Prof. (Dr.) Syed Rais Haider; Dr. Sabiha Kazmi; Dr. Mohd. Zahid Rizvi**
*ISBN:* **978-81-959169-2-4**
*Edition:* **2023**
*Published by:* **Discovery Publishing House, New Delhi (India)**

# Biotic, Abiotic and Ecological factors of Song River

**Rakesh Pant, Bharat Rohilla, *Nirmal Patrick, Amit Gupta**

## ABSTRACT

*Water occurs as a liquid on planet's surface under normal circumstances, making it crucial for conveyance, recreation, and as a habitation for a diversity of flora and fauna. Water molecules have a basic structure (HO), but their physiochemical properties are exceedingly complicated. However it is classic to see ice cubes floating in a glass of cold water, such action is rare for chemical entities. Water's ability to serve as polar solvent changes as it is subjected to increased temperature and pressure. The molecules appear to be more prone to interact with nonpolar molecules as the water temperature rises. Water acts in an unpredictable way beyond its serious temperature and pressure. Beyond its grave point, the difference between the liquid and gaseous forms of water evaporates, and it becomes a volatile liquid, whose density may be altered from liquid to gas by modifying its temperature and pressure. In view of this, our major objective is to study its biotic, abiotic and ecology factors of Song river, Dehradun.*

***Keywords:*** *River ecology, Biotic & Abiotic components, Water chemistry, Song River and Dehradun.*

## INTRODUCTION

Even though the structure of water molecules is simple (HO), the compound's physico-chemical properties are very complicated, & they are not typical of most substances found on earth. Because the solid-state of

**Department of Biotechnology and Department of Life Sciences, Graphic Era (Deemed to be) University, Dehradun-248001 (India)**
***Department of Quality, Eureka Forbes Ltd. Lal Tappar, Dehradun-248140 (India)**

practically every chemical compound is denser than the liquid state, the solid would sink to the bottom of the liquid. The fact that ice floats on the water are very significant in nature because the ice that develops on ponds & lakes in colder climates functions as an insulating barrier, protecting the aquatic life below. Ice developing on a pond would sink if it were denser than liquid water, exposing more water to the chilly temperature. As a result, the pond would ultimately ice over, killing all of the living creatures that were present.

Water molecules have a basic structure (HO), but their physiochemical properties are exceedingly complicated. Although it is common to observe ice cubes floating in a glass of cold water, chemical entities seldom behave in this way. Because almost every chemical compound's solid state is denser than its liquid state, the solid would sink to the bottom of the liquid. If ice formed on ponds were denser than liquid water, it would sink, exposing more water to the cold. As a result, the ponds would eventually freeze over, killing all of the live organisms [3-4].

Water occurs as a liquid on Planet's surface under normal circumstances, making it crucial for conveyance, recreation, & as a habitation for a diversity of flora & fauna. Water's capacity to quickly convert to a vapour allows it to be transported from the sea to inland places, where it precipitate & maintains fauna & flora in the same way that rain does. As of its importance, water has always played a religious and spiritual role in human history. In the 6th century BCE, Thales of Miletus, who is often ascribed with inventing Greek philosophy, felt that water was the single essential building component of substance.

Aristotle, two centuries later, believed water to be one of the 4 elements, alongside earth, air, & fire. For over millennia, water was assumed to be a fundamental substance until research in the late $18^{th}$, discovered that it is a composite made up of the elements hydrogen & oxygen. Filtration & reuse of water are becoming more important as the global populace increases and the need for water rises. Surprisingly, industrial water purity standards are usually greater than those for human use. High-pressure boilers, for example, require water that is at least 99.99 % pure. As saltwater includes significant levels of dissolved salts, it must be distilled for most uses, especially human utilization [3-4].

A single chemical bond connects 2 hydrogen atoms to an oxygen atom in the water molecule. Protons make up the whole nucleus of most hydrogen atoms. Water includes trace quantities of two isotopic forms, deuterium and tritium, which have one & two neutrons in their atomic nuclei, respectively. Deuterium oxide (DO), often known as heavy water, is a neutron moderator used in some nuclear reactors & is important in chemical research. Water has extraordinarily complicated physicochemical properties, despite its basic formula (HO). Its melting point & boiling point is much higher than that of similar substances such as hydrogen sulphide & ammonia. Water is less dense in its solid-state, ice than it is when it is liquid, which is an uncommon feature. The electrical structure of the water molecule is at the base of these irregularities. The molecule of water is curved in an unusual way, rather than being straight. The two hydrogen atoms face the oxygen atom at a 104.5° angle. 95.7 picometres is the OH distance (bond length) (3.77 109 in) (Figure 4.1)

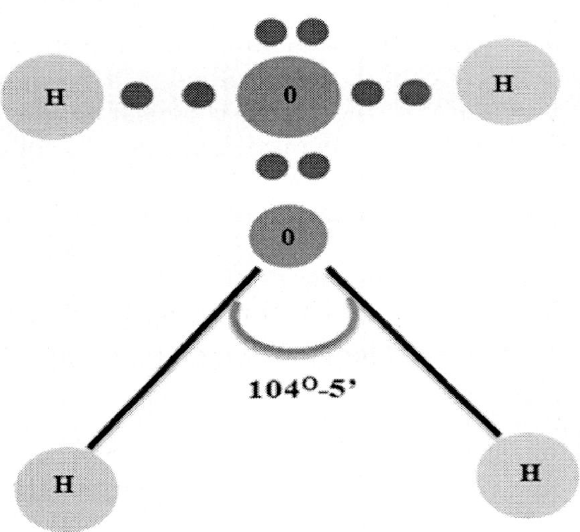


**Fig. 4.1: H and O angle of Aqua molecules**

This means that the hydrogen atoms in one water molecule are drawn to the oxygen atom on the non-bonding electron pairs of the next water molecule. It's considered that liquid water is made up of continually forming & re-forming aggregates of water molecules. This so-called short-range order also explains other noteworthy characteristics of water, such as its increased viscosity & capillary action. An oxygen atom's outer (valence) shell has six electrons and may hold up to eight electrons. An oxygen atom gives up one of its electrons to the nucleus of another atom in return for a fraction of that atom's electron when it creates a single chemical connection. When an oxygen atom is joined to two hydrogen atoms, its outer electron shell is full. The water molecule's electron configuration may be observed here. Each dot represents a non-shared pair of electrons. This situation can also be represented by putting the water molecule in a cube [3-4].

**Physical Properties of Aqua**

Molar Mass: 18.01 g/mole

Melting Point: 32°F

Boiling Point: 212°F

Max Density (@ 3.98 degree Celsius): 1 g/cm^3
Density (@ 25°C): 997 kg/$m^3$
Vapour pressure (@ 25°C): 3.17 Kpa
Heat of fusion (@ 0°C): 6.010 Kj/mol
Heat of vaporization (@100°C): 40.63KJ $mol^{-1}$
Heat of formation (@ 25°C): 285.9 KJ $mole^{-1}$
Entropy of vaporization (@ 25°C): 118.8 J/° C moles
Viscosity: 0.8903 centipoise
Surface tension (25°C): 71.97 dynes/cm

## RIVER ECOLOGY

The ecology of a stream relates to the interactions of living organisms with one another and with their surroundings, which is referred to as the ecosystem. An ecosystem is the sum of interactions between flora, fauna, and microorganisms, and between them and non-living physiochemical components, in a specific natural area. One of the most familiar example is seen in Song river as shown in figure 4.2.

- River environments are characterized by primarily unidirectional water flow.
- A constant state of physical change.
- There are numerous microhabitats.
- Water flow rates have a lot of variation.
- Plants and animals have evolved to exist in low-flow environments.

## ABIOTIC COMPONENTS

**Water Flow-** The key characteristic that distinguishes river ecology from other water ecosystems is the flow of water. Water flow intensity ranges from raging rapids to gentle backwaters. Water has a variable speed and is vulnerable to chaotic turbulence. Snowmelt, rain, and groundwater all have the potential to disrupt the flow. Through erosion and sedimentation, water movement may change the morphology of riverbeds, resulting in a range of different environments [1-2]. One of the example is seen in Song river, Lacchiwala, Uttarakhand (Figure 4.3).

**Temperature-** The temperature of water in rivers fluctuates depending on the surrounding environment; as a result, the temperature is an important abiotic element for them. Temperature variations between the surface & the bottom of deep, slow-moving rivers can be substantial. Water temperature is affected by a variety of factors including climate, shade, and elevation. Poikilotherms are species that live in these types of habitats, and their internal temperature fluctuates to fit their surroundings [1, 2-4].

Seasonal changes are most intense in the arctic, desert, and temperate systems, which display large diurnal oscillations. The temperature of lotic systems can be influenced by the amount of shade, weather, and terrain [2-5].

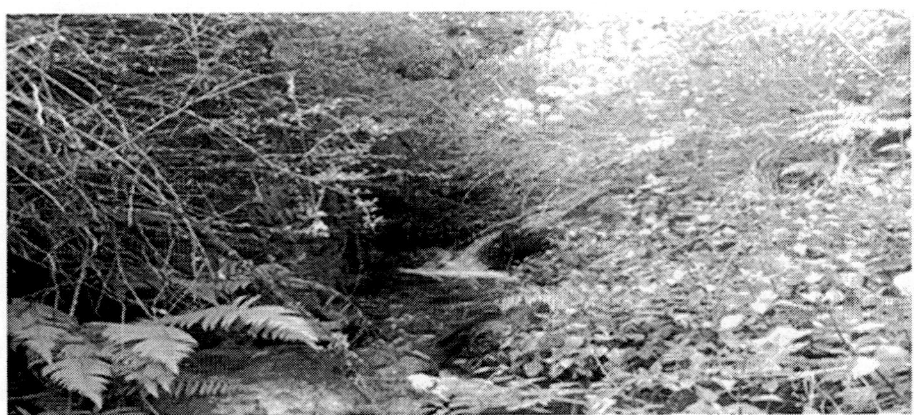

Song River Uniyal Gaon, Uttarakhand, India Site

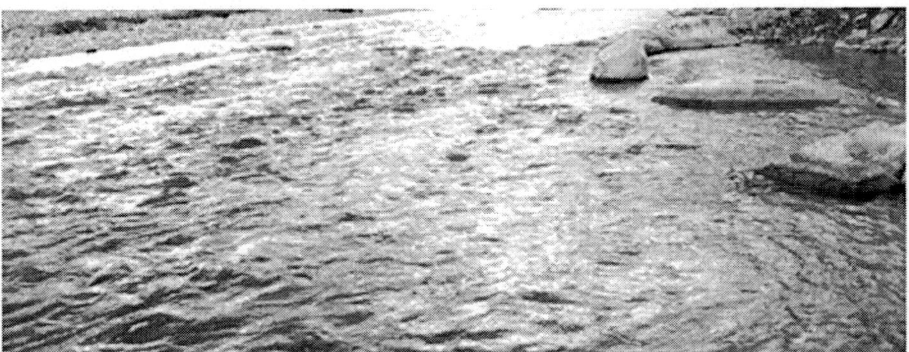

Song River Dawara, Uttarakhand, India Site

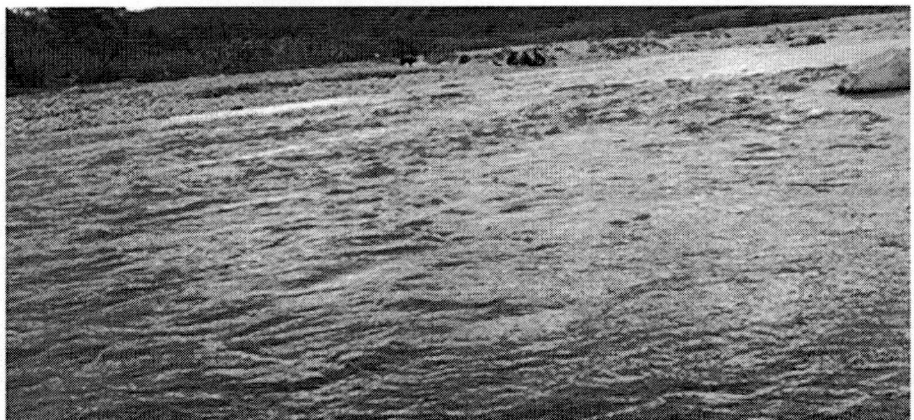

Song River Raipur, Uttarakhand, India Site

**Fig. 4.2: Song River**

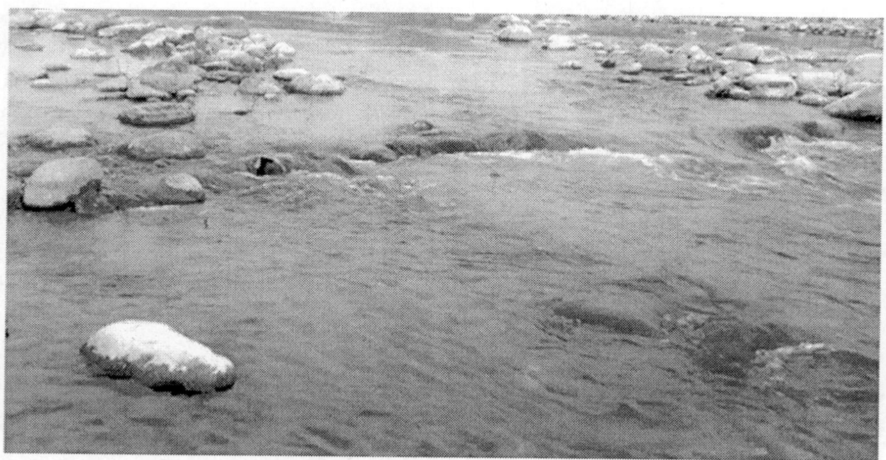

**Fig. 4.3: Song River Lacchiwala, Uttarakhand, India Site**

**Chemical properties-** The water chemistry differs from one river environment to the next. Rain & pollutants from human sources can also impact it. It is generally governed by inputs from the nearby ecosystem/ local region but it can also be changed by rain & the inclusion of contamination from human sources. Most species require oxygen to survive; hence it is the major significant chemical ingredient of drainage systems. It usually enters the water at the surface, but as the water temp increases, its solvent declines. Fast, turbulent waters expose a larger portion of the water surface to the air and have lower temperatures, allowing for increased oxygen intake than calm backwaters. If water circulation is low, animal activity is excessive, or there is a lot of organic waste in the river, oxygen is restricted.

The number of dissolved solutes and gases present in the water column of a stream ecosystem affects the aqua chemistry. Apart from the water itself, river water can comprise a variety of things.

- Significant ions and dissolved inorganic matter.
- Inorganic nutrients dissolved.
- Organic matter gases, both suspended and dissolved.
- Pollutants and trace metals.

## BIOTIC COMPONENTS

The biotic components of a habitat are the live elements. Rivers are home to a diverse range of biotic species, which includes microbes, primary producers, & other invertebrates, as well as fish and other vertebrates.

**Biofilm-** A biofilm is a film formed by seaweed, fungus, microbes, and other microscopic microorganisms that live in a river bottom or benthos. Biofilms are most significant biological interkinesis in stream habitat, & perhaps the most important in intermittent rivers, because the water column is less essential during lengthy times of low activity in the water processes. They are autotrophic and heterotrophic microbial communities that dwell in a matrix of hydrated extracellular polymeric molecules (EPS). Biofilms are therefore a highly active biological consortium, capable of using both organic & inorganic resources from the aqueous phase, as well as light and chemical sources of energy. The physical structure of biofilms, as well as the adaptability of the organisms that live inside them, ensure & maintain their survival in difficult situations or when environs factors change. Biofilm layers were present in several areas of the Song River such as Raipur, Doiwala, Kansrao, Chiddarwala, Nepali Farm (Figure 4.4) [6-7].

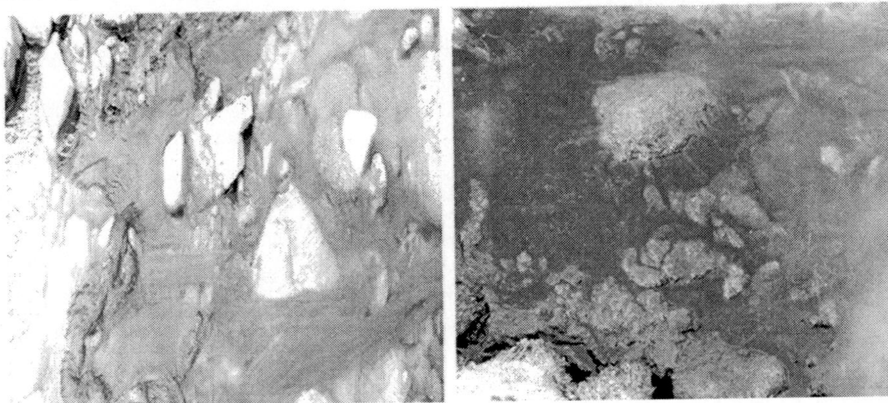

**Fig. 4.4: Biofilm in Song River Dwara, Uttarakhand, India Site**

**Microbes-** Microbes can be found in abundance in flowing water. Microbes break down organic matter into inorganic molecules that plants and other microorganisms may utilise. Bacteria plays major part in the recycling. On testing the water of the Song River (Figure 4.5), the *Enterobacteriaceae* family microorganisms were found [1-7].

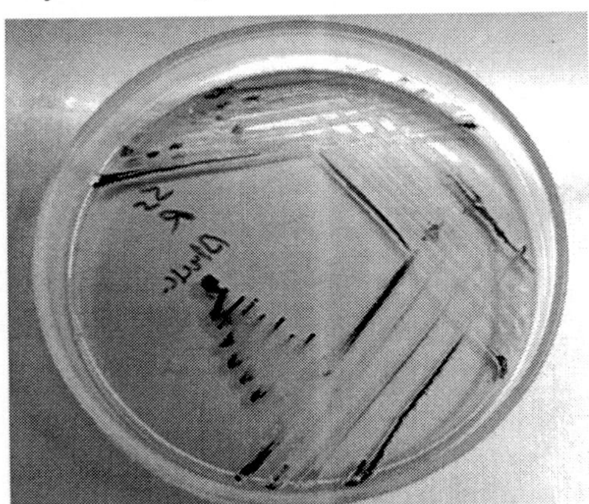

**Fig. 4.5: Song River Salmonella microbe isolated plate**

**Primary producers-** The major important origins of main production in most brooks and waterways are algae, which include phytoplankton and periphyton. Because phytoplankton floats freely in the water column, colonies in fast-moving streams cannot be sustained. Slow-moving rivers & backwaters, on the other hand, may support large populations. The River Song yielded a total of 27 phytoplankton genera, divided into three classes, seven orders, & twenty-one families. The key classes were *Chlorophyceae, Bacillariophyceae,* and *Myxophyceae.* The biggest category of phytoplankton was 13 genera of *Chlorophyceae* (green algae), followed by 12 genera of *Bacillariophyceae* and 2 genera of *Myxophyceae* (blue-green algae). The significant *Chlorophyceae* and *Bacillariophyceae* species richness seen in the lower Ebro River might be regarded as freshwater ecosystem features. Plants have limited adaptations to rapid flow and thrive best in slower currents. Mosses & liverworts, for example, are more primitive plants that adhere themselves to solid surfaces (Figure 4.6). This is more common in cooler headwaters, where the stony ground provides attachment points [3-5].

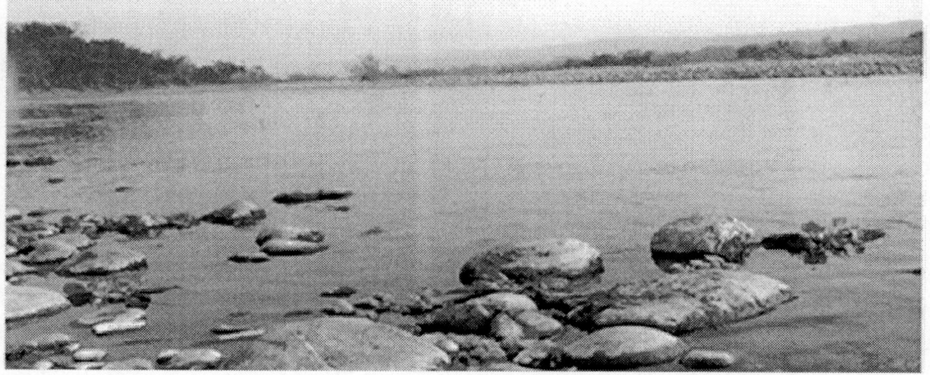

**Fig. 4.6: Primary producers in Song River Kansrao, Uttarakhand, India Site**

**Fish and other invertebrates-** The most well-known residents of perennial flowing water are fish. The capacity of a species of fishes to exist in running waters is determined by its swimming speed & the length of time it can sustain that pace. This ability varies widely between species & is dependent on the environment in which it can thrive. Because constant swimming consumes lot of energy, fish only stay in the stream for brief periods of time. There are various species of fishes found in the Song River (Figure 4.7) such as *Clarias batrachus, Schistura savona, Esomus danricus, Labeo dyocheilus, Cyprinus carpio,* etc. [5-7].

Crawfish, leeches, insects, flatworms, crustaceans and molluscs found in streams are examples of invertebrates, which lack a backbone or spine. They can be found on sea surface, on & under boulders, in or below the substratum, or floating in the current in practically every accessible habitat.

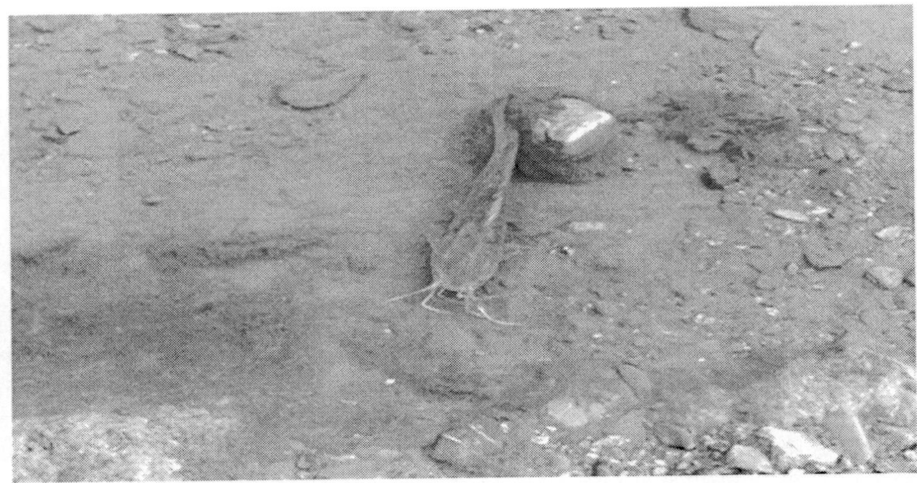

**Fig. 4.7: Invertebrates in Song River Raipur, Uttarakhand, India Site**

**Habitat Loss-** Important river and floodplain ecosystems can be degraded or destroyed as a result of human activity. Hard shorelines, for example, increase water velocity, hastening erosion and harming fish populations. Digging channels or straightening rivers causes flooding by destroying neighbouring floodplains and wetlands. The loss of shelter from river development can result in warmer waters, putting numerous species at risk. Polluted runoff from streets, parking lots, and rooftops is also increased by paved surfaces. Long before they reach the sea, overused rivers can dry up, eliminating crucial ecosystems.

**Polluted Runoff-** Fertilizers, herbicides, & pesticides can pollute rivers and streams due to outdated farming techniques. Excess nutrients & hazardous chemicals can then build up in rivers, resulting in algal blooms and "dead zones" where aquatic life cannot live.

Storm water and sewage systems that are combined can overflow, dumping untreated human waste into rivers. These spills pose a health concern and contribute to nutrient contamination. The ensuing algal bloom can be harmful to both fish & humans.

In the Song River, there were lots of plastic bottles, discarded clothes, and wood debris was found everywhere (Figure 4.8). In some places, there was in large quantity and in some less. [8-10]

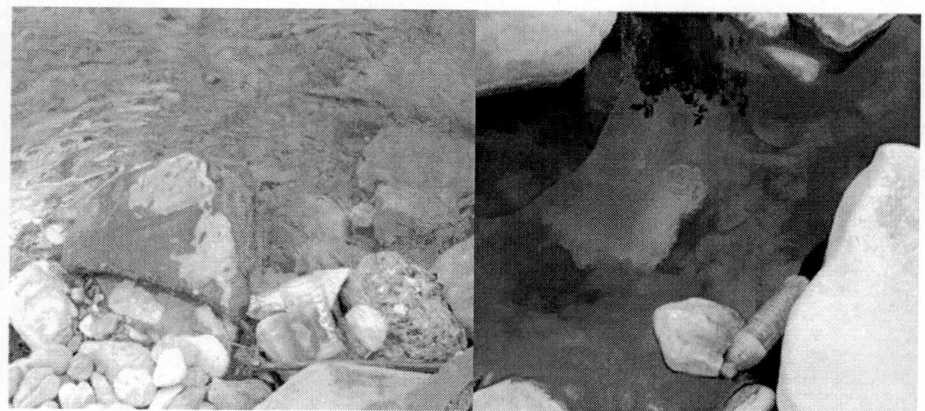

**Fig. 4.8: Song River Maldevta & Dwara, Uttarakhand, India Site**

## REFERENCES


1. Khanna, D.R., Singh, V., Bhutiani, R., Chandra, K.S., Matta, G. and Kumar, D. (2007). A Study of Biotic and Abiotic Factors of Song River at Dehradun, Uttarakhand. Environment Conservation Journal; 8 (3): pp. 117-126.
2. Ranal, D., Gupta, S.K. and Rana, R. Fish Fauna of Doon Valley, District Dehradun, Uttarakhand, India. International Journal of Advanced Research in Biological Sciences 2017; 4 (12): pp.120-132.
3. https://www.britannica.com/science/water.pp.1-13.
4. https://www.britannica.com/science/hydrosphere/Congruent-and-incongruent weathering-reactions. pp. 1-11.
5. Chalotra, S. and Rauthan, J.V.S. (2017). Bio-Diversity of Phytoplankton of Song River in Doon Valley, Uttarakhand. Review of Research; 6(12): pp. 1-6.
6. Singh, D., Rana, J.S. and Seyiekuolie. Water Quality and Assemblages of Phytoplankton Communities of River Song in the Lower Himalaya. International Journal of Water Research 2017; 7(2): pp. 39-47.
7. Kim, J.S, Seo, W. Il and Baek D. Seasonally varying effects of Environmental Factors on Phytoplankton Abundance in the regulated Rivers. Scientific Reports 2019; 9 (266): pp. 1-12.
8. https://www.thoughtco.com/definition-of-water-in-chemistry-605946.pp.1-3.
9. Bhutiani, R. and Khanna, D.R. (2007). Ecological Study of River Suswa: Modelling DO and BOD. Environ Monit Assess; 125: pp.183-195.
10. Bhutiani, R., Khanna, D.R. and Rawat, S. (2014). Recent Trend in Physico-Chemical Parameters of Song River at Nepali Farm District Dehradun, Uttarakhand, India. International Journal of Researches in Biosciences, Agriculture and Technology; 2(2): pp. 34-44.


**Corresponding author: Dr. Amit Gupta, Associate Professor, Department of Biotechnology, Graphic Era (Deemed to be) University, Dehradun, India.**
**Email id: dr.amitgupta.bt@geu.ac.in**

Pages: 34-39
**Emerging Environmental Contaminants and Global Healthcare Systems**
*Editors:* **Prof. (Dr.) Shyam Narain Pandey; Murtaza Abid**
**Prof. (Dr.) Syed Rais Haider; Dr. Sabiha Kazmi; Dr. Mohd. Zahid Rizvi**
*ISBN:* **978-81-959169-2-4**
*Edition:* **2023**
*Published by:* **Discovery Publishing House, New Delhi (India)**

# The Impact of Environmental Toxins on the Cardivascular System

**Khushi Kashyap and Amit Gupta**

## ABSTRACT

*In literature, exposure of environmental toxins may become as one of the major global health issue all over the world. This may happen due to enhancement in industrial and sewage waste, pesticides used in agriculture, waste water etc. which directly targets the health of animals including human. Now the risk of disease may be increased by exposure to pollutants and chemicals. Among all, pollution (e.g. air, water, soil etc.) is the most significant environmental factor that causes cardiovascular disease. Actually, its mechanism of action may totally have varied in case of metals, the only way to eliminate from the body with the help of biomarkers to detect its early signs of this cardiovascular disease. So, there is a strong link between pollution and an elevated risk of cardiovascular illness and mortality. In this chapter, we focused on impact of environmental toxins on the cardiovascular system.*

**Keywords:** *Environmental toxins; cardiovascular system; pollution and risk.*

## INTRODUCTION

One of the most leading cause of death worldwide i.e. Cardiovascular disease with increasingly mortality rate. Traditionally, disease is mainly caused through poor diet, obesity, lacking of physical fitness etc. and also causing disease from the environment through pollution. For the last thirteen years (1990-2013), there is sudden enhancement (41 percent) in cardiovascular cases worldwide and trend is still going on. The major reason

**Department of Biotechnology, Graphic Era (Deemed to be) University, Dehradun, (India)**

for enhancement of cases because of low and middle income countries and these countries are not being able to prevent the burden of these communicable diseases e.g. malaria and influenza [1, 2]. In this regard, various efforts from government and private agencies were taken into consideration for declining in cardiovascular mortality rate i.e. generate awareness around people to banned smoking, improvement in medical services, improved physical activity etc. In contrast, another important factor i.e. environmental toxins may directly target the cardiovascular (e.g. heart) system. In simple words, environmental toxins mean those substances which may directly target or disrupt our health because of poisonous (i.e. chemicals and compounds) substances that disrupt or alter immunobiological processes, and these organisms may be responsible for causing disease. The most familiar example is seen in case of heart and its vascular system where environmental toxins (i.e. heavy metals, pollution etc.) may cause structural damage in heart and also disturbed or altered its functional properties i.e. electrical conduction system abnormalities, declining in cardiac output etc [3-5]. In this regard, successful treatment may be required for removal of the toxic agent and, in some cases, treatment with a known as antidote. In view of this, various conferences related to Heart and Toxins which brings together some leading scientists from around the world to share the most up-to-date research and clinical trials on the link between genetic vulnerability, gene expression, and environmental factors in cardiovascular disease. Also, there have been statistically significant links found between particle air pollution and ischemic heart disease, arrhythmias, and heart failure. An increased risk of cardiovascular disease and coronary heart disease has been associated to arsenic, lead, cadmium, and copper exposure. These effects have been attributed to changes in the production or reactivity of nitric oxide, which may be caused by ambient oxidants or increased endogenous formation of reactive oxygen species [6, 7]. Drug, toxin, and infection exposure during pregnancy has been associated to heart birth abnormalities and early Cardiovascular disease later in life. As a result, many people think about Cardiovascular disease as a reaction to environmental threats. Heart disease is caused by complicated interplay between genes and the environment. Also, Human research, in contrast to animal studies, reveal that both pulmonary and systemic alterations may play a role in the cardiovascular effects of PM, and that underlying illness is a potent modifier of the total response. According to studies, occupational exposure to butadiene, vinyl chloride or formaldehyde or chemicals used by undertakers, embalmers, and perfumery workers, increases Cardiovascular disease risk, bolster the relationship between Cardiovascular disease and volatile chemical exposure. As a result, it's critical to determine how much people are exposed to volatile and non-volatile contaminants in their microenvironment and to build personal monitors that accurately and faithfully reflect individual exposures in real time [8-10].

## FACTORS IN THE ENVIRONMENT THAT CAN CAUSE HEART DISEASE AND STROKE

- **Drinking Water [11, 12]**
  - *Lead:*

    Blood pressure can be raised by lead poisoning. While the majority of individuals are exposed to lead through paint particles, it is also found in drinking water.
  - *Arsenic:*

    Long-term exposure to high levels of arsenic, a naturally occurring metal found in some sections of the country's drinking water, can cause heart disease.
  - *Excessive Heat Events:*

    People who have had a heart attack or a stroke have weakened cooling mechanisms, making them more exposed to heat. Certain drugs, such as antidepressants and circulatory meds, can make people more vulnerable to heat incidents.
- **Indoor Air Pollution [13]**

  Second hand smoking, cleaning product odours, and even carbon monoxide can all be found in indoor air.

  These indoor contaminants can be extremely deadly, especially for people who are at risk of stroke or heart disease.

  ❑ *Smoke:*

  Smoking is known to cause heart disease and stroke, but inhaling the same amount of second hand smoke and active smoking smoke is just as harmful.

  Small carbon particles can be found in the smoke from wood-burning stoves and fireplaces. In elderly people with heart problems, these particles can induce chest pain and palpitations, as well as shortness of breath and weariness.

  ❑ *Household Products:*

  Cleaning products, paint solvents, and pesticide vapours all require good ventilation and minimal exposure to avoid negative consequences.
  - Paint solvent fumes such as mineral spirits, turpentine, methanol, and xylene, put a strain on the lungs and heart, cause irregular pulse.
  - Paint chips or dust produced at the time of renovations, can cause major health problems, such as high blood pressure.
  - Toxic fumigants and insecticides are frequently the source of pesticide poisoning. Arrhythmia or a very sluggish pulse are common signs of this form of poisoning.

- Exposure can cause a heart attack or even death in the most extreme circumstances.

❑ ***Carbon Monoxide:***

It is a colourless and odourless gas that is difficult to detect also a deadly contaminant. It is especially dangerous for patients who have heart disease, clogged arteries, or congestive heart failure since it reduces the blood's ability to transport oxygen.

- **Outdoor Air Pollution [14]**

❑ ***Particle Pollution***

Small soot particles found in outdoor air can be harmful, and persons with heart disease, chronic obstructive pulmonary disease, and asthma are at the greatest risk. Vehicles, power plants, industrial smokestacks, and fires are only few of the sources of particles. Some particles are directly discharged into the atmosphere, while others are formed as a result of complex chemical interactions in the atmosphere. Particles can travel hundreds to thousands of kilometres downwind, affecting people who are thousands of miles away from the source.

❑ ***Pollutant Gases***

Ozone, sulphur dioxide, and other pollutant gases components like nitrogen dioxide are also important and have been linked to detrimental health effects as a result of air pollution. Ozone is a strong irritant to the skin, lungs, and airways, causing chest pain and also misinterpreted as a heart attack too.

## SYNOPSIS OF THE CASE STUDY

Heart disease, the nation's biggest cause of death, and stroke, the third most common cause of death, cost the country hundreds of billions of dollars each year. According to the CDC, heart disease killed 652,091 people in 2005, accounting for 27.1 percent of all fatalities in the United States.

## STEPS THAT CAN BE PERFORMED TO REDUCE THE RISK OF HEAT DISEASE AND STROKE [15, 16]

- Encourage your municipal government to act.
- Local governments should make some modest measures to avert hazards and inform older people about the safeguards available to them.
- The greatest method to avoid heart disease and stroke is to live a healthy lifestyle.
- Furthermore, older persons should restrict their exposure to risk factors in the environment.

- Take frequent fresh air breaks while painting and remain out of painted rooms for several days.
- Avoid carbon monoxide poisoning.
- Avoid smoke from tobacco
- Visit your doctor on a regular basis to have your blood pressure, diabetes, and hyperlipidemia (excess lipids in the bloodstream) checked and treated.

So, these findings showed its importance of environmental toxins in enhancing the burden of cardiovascular disease. These steps may have a key policy implication given that current global noncommunicable disease prevention strategies (eg, WHO 2018 Report) are focused primarily on tackling behavioural determinants.

## CONCLUSION

In short, exposure of environmental toxins which is directly associated with cardiovascular disease and coronary heart disease. In view of this, firstly, we identified the specific environmental toxin or factor which is closely linked or associated with cardiovascular (heart) disease. So, it may be possible to discriminate between processes and genes that respond to environmental perturbations and those that contribute directly to disease development. Furthermore, by studying cardiovascular reactions in real-world situations, we may be able to learn more about how cardiovascular disease develops in real-world settings and how it might be prevented and eased rather than just treated symptomatically.

## REFERENCES

1. GBD 2016 Disease and Injury Incidence and Prevalence Collaborators. Global, Regional, and National Incidence, Prevalence, and years lived with Disability for 328 Diseases and Injuries for 195 Countries, 1990-2016: A Systematic Analysis for the Global Burden of Disease Study 2016. Lancet 2017; 390: 1211-1259.
2. Li, Z., Ma, Z., van der Kuijp, T.J., Yuan, Z. and Huang, L. A Review of Soil Heavy Metal Pollution from Mines in China: Pollution and Health Risk Assessment. Sci Total Environ 2014; 468-469: 843-53.
3. Jomova, K., Jenisova, Z., Feszterova, M., *et al*. Arsenic: Toxicity, Oxidative Stress and Human Disease. J Appl Toxicol 2011; 31: 95-107.
4. Tellez-Plaza, M., Jones, M.R., Dominguez-Lucas, A., Guallar, E. and Navas-Acien, A. Cadmium Exposure and Clinical Cardiovascular Disease: A Systematic Review. Curr Atheroscler Rep 2013; 15: 356.
5. Navas-Acien, A., Guallar, E., Silbergeld, E.K. and Rothenberg, S.J. Lead Exposure and Cardiovascular Disease— A Systematic Review. Environ Health Perspect 2007; 115: 472-82.
6. Navas-Acien, A., Sharrett, A.R., Silbergeld EK, *et al*. Arsenic Exposure and Cardiovascular Disease: A Systematic Review of the Epidemiologic Evidence. Am J Epidemiol 2005; 162: 1037-49.

7. Bhatnagar A. Environmental Cardiology: Studying Mechanistic Links between Pollution, and Heart Disease. Circ Res 2006; 99: 692-705.
8. Chen, Y., Graziano, J.H., Parvez, F., *et al.* Arsenic Exposure from Drinking Water and Mortality from Cardiovascular Disease in Bangladesh: Prospective Cohort Study. BMJ 2011; 342: d2431.
9. Farzan, S.F., Chen, Y., Rees, J.R., Zens, M.S. and Karagas, M.R. Risk of Death from Cardiovascular Disease Associated with Low-level Arsenic exposure among Long-term Smokers in a US Population-based Study. Toxicol Appl Pharmacol 2015; 287: 93-7.
10. Wade, T.J., Xia, Y., Mumford, J., *et al.* Cardiovascular Disease and Arsenic Exposure in Inner Mongolia, China: A Case Control Study. Environ Health 2015; 12: 14-35.
11. Garland, M., Morris, J.S., Rosner, B.A., *et al.* Toenail Trace Element Levels as Biomarkers: Reproducibility over a 6-year period. Cancer Epidemiol Biomarkers Prev 1993; 2: 493-7.
12. Ekong, E.B., Jaar, B.G. and Weaver, V.M. Lead-related Nephrotoxicity: A Review of the Epidemiologic Evidence. Kidney Int 2006; 70: 2074-84.
13. Tong, S., Von Schirnding, Y.E. and Prapamontol, T. Environmental Lead Exposure: A public Health Problem of Global Dimensions. Bull World Health Organ 2000; 78: 1068-77.
14. Muntner, P., Menke, A., DeSalvo, K.B., Rabito, F.A. and Batuman, V. Continued Decline in Blood Lead Levels Among Adults in the United States: The National Health and Nutrition Examination Surveys. Arch Intern Med 2005; 165: 2155-61.
15. Shiue, I. Higher Urinary Heavy Metal, Arsenic, and Phthalate Concentrations in people with High Blood Pressure: US NHANES, 2009-2010. Blood Press 2014; 23: 363-9.
16. Abhyankar, L.N., Jones, M.R., Guallar, E. and Navas-Acien, A. Arsenic Exposure and Hypertension: A Systematic Review. Environ Health Perspect 2012; 120: 494-500.

**Corresponding author: Dr. Amit Gupta, Associate Professor, Department of Biotechnology, Graphic Era (Deemed to be) University, Dehradun, India.**
**Email id: dr.amitgupta.bt@geu.ac.in**

Pages: 40-47

**Emerging Environmental Contaminants and Global Healthcare Systems**

*Editors:* **Prof. (Dr.) Shyam Narain Pandey; Murtaza Abid**
**Prof. (Dr.) Syed Rais Haider; Dr. Sabiha Kazmi; Dr. Mohd. Zahid Rizvi**

*ISBN:* **978-81-959169-2-4**

*Edition:* **2023**

*Published by:* **Discovery Publishing House, New Delhi (India)**

# Effect of Environmental Factors and Climate Change *Mycobacterium Tuberculosis*

**Khushi Kashyap and Amit Gupta**

## ABSTRACT

*Mycobacterium tuberculosis infects around one-third of the world's population, making it one of the most effective human diseases. At least nine Mycobacterium tuberculosis species are known to cause human tuberculosis and zoonotic disease. Mycobacterium tuberculosis sensu stricto is the bacterium that causes the vast majority of human tuberculosis cases worldwide. The bacteria are assumed to have descended from a single clonal ancestor, with 99.9% sequence identity. Furthermore, studies published in journals addressing tuberculosis in Malaysia as a result of environmental factors show that the environment is a risk factor for the disease. As a result, the purpose of this study is to collect data on tuberculosis in individuals, including its forms, prevention, and case studies.*

**Keywords:** *Mycobacterium tuberculosis; bacteria; environmental and prevention.*

## INTRODUCTION

Pollution is defined as any substance or form of energy released into the environment faster than it can be dispersed, diluted, decomposed, recycled, or safely stored. According to the environment, the three main types of pollution are air pollution, water pollution, and land contamination. In today's culture, specific sorts of pollution, such as noise, light, and plastic pollution, are also a cause of concern. Pollution, in any form, can be harmful

**Department of Biotechnology, Graphic Era (Deemed to be) University, Dehradun, (India)**

to the environment, wildlife, and human health and well-being. In general, shortness of breath, coughing, wheezing, asthma attacks, and chest pain are all signs of inflamed airways caused by pollution (1, 2). In addition, lung cancer, consumption, heart attacks, strokes, and, in the worst-case scenario, early mortality are all linked to air pollution exposure. This disease is considered as one of the most serious public health issue in India. In some countries, TB disease has already been reduced to less than 10 cases and 1 death per 100,000 people.

Between 2001 and 2020, India's tuberculosis fatality rate decreased slightly, from 57 cases per 100,000 people in 2001 to 32 cases per 100,000 in 2020. With an estimated 220,000 deaths each year, According to a case study conducted at a New York hospital, 591 out of 651 people who were screened finished the initial assessment. Tuberculosis infection was found to be prevalent in 41% of the sample. Infection risk factors included being born outside of the United States, living in a communal setting, and taking drugs. Human immunodeficiency virus (HIV) infection was not a risk factor for infection but there were also eleven active tuberculosis cases were discovered. The great majority of tuberculosis patients were HIV-positive or at high risk of being infected (3-5).

In literature, environmental factors such as weather and air pollution which showed a significant correlation with tuberculosis occurrence. The "tubercle bacillus" is another name for *M. tuberculosis*. It is a pathogenic bacterium that belongs to the *Mycobacteriaceae* family and was discovered by Robert Koch in 1882 (6, 7). Tuberculosis, often known as consumption, is a bacterial infection that affects the lungs. *Mycobacterium tuberculosis* is the microorganism that causes tuberculosis. Tuberculosis is a disease that affects the lungs, but it can also affect the kidneys, spine, and brain. It's a bacterial infection that can be both acute and persistent. Infection spreads mostly by airborne droplets inhaled by a person afflicted with tuberculosis. Bacteria cause Tubercles, which are tiny tissue lumps caused by bacteria. *Bacillus subtilis* belongs to the high G+C bacteria, which are Gram Positive Bacteria that constitute a monophyletic group within the low G+C bacteria (8, 9). Two types of tuberculosis disease (10) are reported (Figure 6.1)

- *Latent tuberculosis:* The germs of tuberculosis are present in the body but remain dormant. However, when a condition such as HIV or diabetes was present, the TB bacteria became active.
- *Active tuberculosis:* The germs proliferate, making a person unwell and increasing the risk of disease spread. Adults with latent tuberculosis account for 90% of active cases.

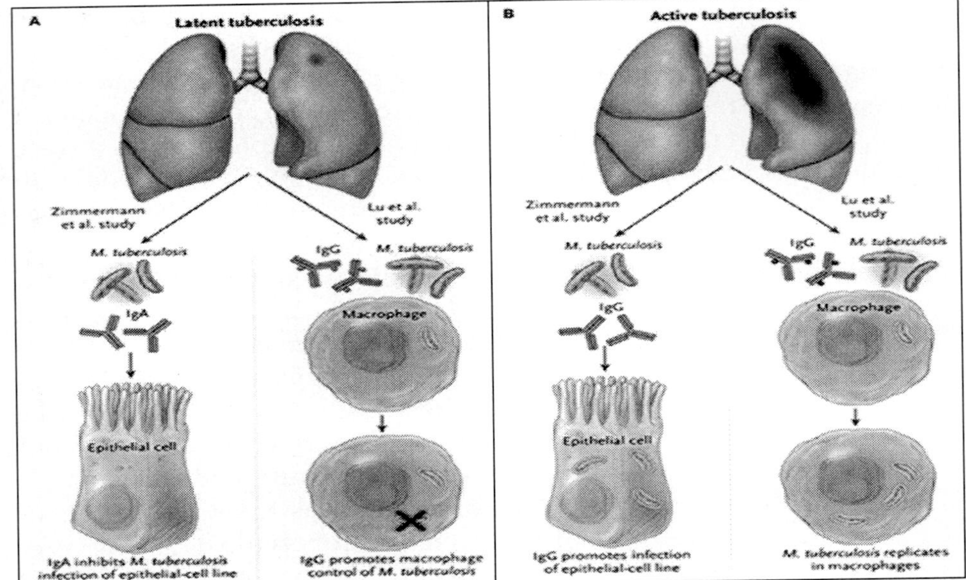


**Fig. 6.1: Latent and active TB**

*Mycobacterium tuberculosis immunological lifespan, as well as the disease's progression-Mycobacterium tuberculosis* is usually delivered by aerosol, and the innate immune response serves as a first line of defence in the alveolar region. *Mycobacterium tuberculosis* can be readily removed in the early stages of infection. The spread of infection and the activation of the adaptive immune response are both aided by the migration of antigen-presenting cells to lymph nodes [11, 12]. *Mycobacterium tuberculosis* granulomas are regulated by T-lymphocytes, resulting in latent tuberculosis infection (LTBI). Latent tuberculosis becomes active when the immune balance between the host and the pathogen is broken. The patient is developing symptoms at this point and is at danger of infecting others. (Figure 6.2)

The bacterium that causes tuberculosis is transmitted from one person to another through the air. When a person with TB of the lungs or throat coughs, talks, or sings, the germs are released into the air [13]. Others in the proximity may be sickened if they breath the infection (Figure 6.3).

When a huge amount of any chemical or type of energy is released into the environment quicker than it can be dispersed or securely stored, it is referred to be pollution. Both manmade and natural materials that are formed, used, and disposed in an unsustainable manner are referred to as pollution. Pollution has a multitude of harmful health effects on humans. As a result, this study looks into the effects of environmental elements and climate change on human health, particularly lung disease, such as tuberculosis (TB).

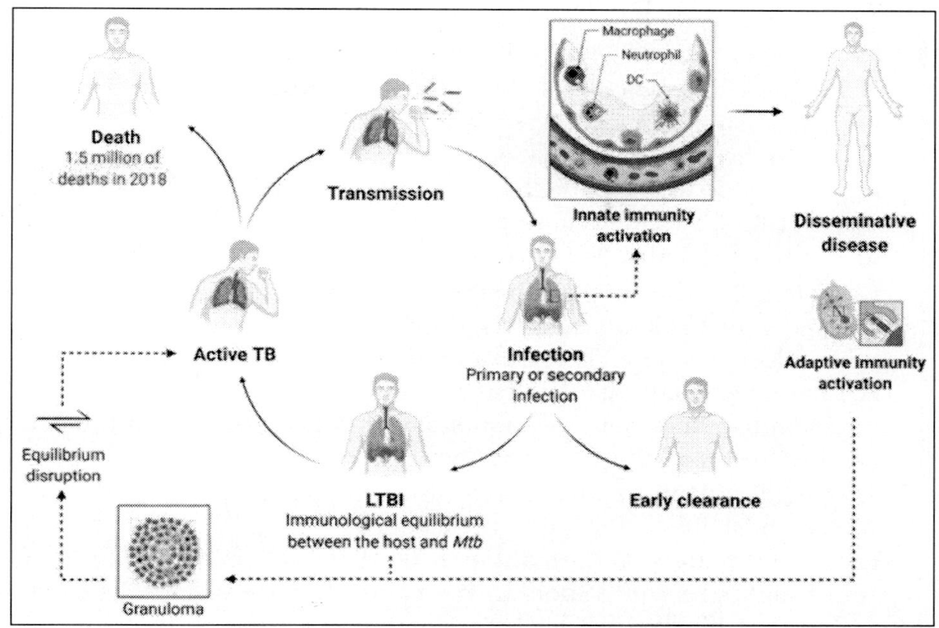


**Fig. 6.2: Transmission of Mycobacterium tuberculosis (Mtb) through aerosol**

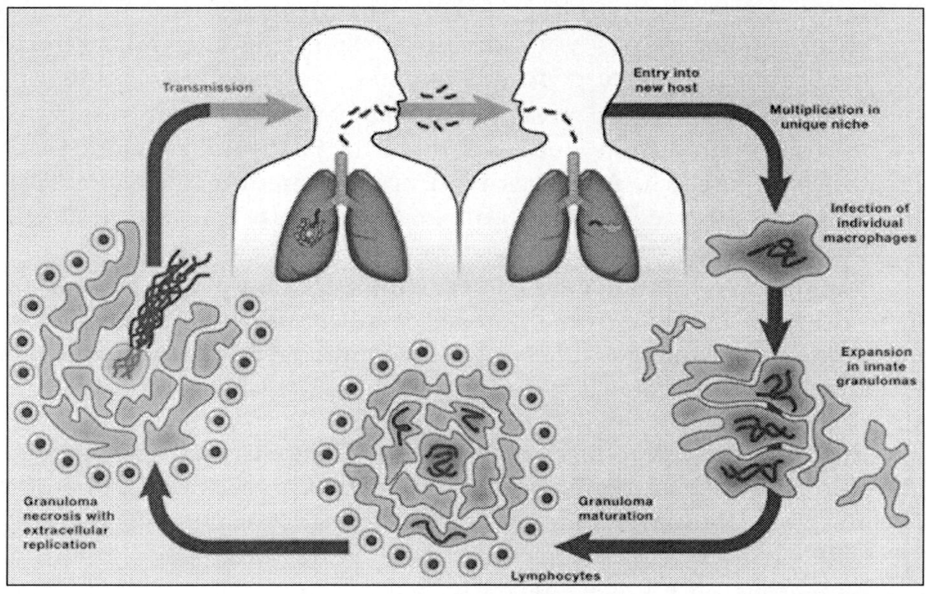


**Fig. 6.3: The diagram depicts the spread of tuberculosis in a specific human body**

There are several tests for tuberculosis detection, including skin tests, blood tests, imaging tests, and sputum tests [14-16].

- *Skin Test:* The tuberculosis skin test is not without flaws. It can give the impression that someone has tuberculosis when they don't. It may also give the impression that a person does not have tuberculosis when in fact they do. If the patient has recently received the Bacille Calmette-Guerin (BCG) vaccine, a false-positive result is possible. It's also possible to get unexpectedly bad results.
- *Blood Test:* Blood testing can be used to confirm or rule out tuberculosis. These tests look at how the body's immune system reacts to tuberculosis bacteria. These examinations just require one office visit. A blood test may be useful if the individual is at high risk of TB infection but does not have a positive skin test result, or if the person has just received the BCG vaccine.
- *Imaging Test:* If the patient's skin test comes back positive, the doctor would most likely prescribe a chest X-ray or a CT scan. This could reveal pulmonary abnormalities caused by active tuberculosis, or it could highlight white spots in the patient's lungs where the immune system has blocked TB bacteria from entering the body.
- *Sputum Test:* If a chest X-ray shows signs of tuberculosis, a sample of sputum, the mucus that comes up when a patient cough, may be obtained. The samples are tested for tuberculosis bacteria. Sputum samples can also be used to screen for drug-resistant tuberculosis strains. This assists your doctor in selecting the most effective medications. These tests' results can take four to eight weeks to arrive.
- In addition, one of the most often utilised machine learning approaches in disease prediction studies is the artificial neural network (ANN). In a few research, ANN has been used to predict Tuberculosis cases. In terms of prediction accuracy, the results showed that ANN performed the best.

Population relocation happens as extreme climatic events become more often, resulting in a rise in the number of tuberculosis-vulnerable and risk populations. It encourages tuberculosis transmission and active tuberculosis development while also disturbing tuberculosis diagnosis and treatment. Also, at low humidity, the link between humidity and tuberculosis is strong and quick, but the risk reduces as the lag lengthens. The risk of tuberculosis (TB) is greatest during periods of low temperature, low humidity, and low rainfall, when the optimal weather conditions correspond to the lowest risk of infection.

Numerous efforts were taken by various researchers and doctors in order to control the burden of this disease. In this regard, 6-month treatment programme can successfully treat 85% of persons with tuberculosis disease, and 1–6-month pharmaceutical regimens can be used to treat TB infection. Universal health coverage (UHC) is necessary to ensure that everyone who is afflicted with a disease or illness has access to treatment. Poverty, malnutrition, HIV infection, smoking, and diabetes are all TB-related factors that can be addressed by multi-sectoral interventions, lowering the number of people who become infected and develop disease [16, 17].

1. BCG vaccination
2. Early diagnostics
3. Environmental factors can reduce the spread of tuberculosis:
   - Good ventilation: Because tuberculosis can persist in the air for several hours if there is no ventilation, good ventilation is essential.
   - Natural light: UV light kills tuberculosis bacteria in the natural world.
   - Good hygiene: Cover your lips and nose when coughing or sneezing to prevent tuberculosis bacteria from spreading.

## HOW DOES THE ENVIRONMENT AFFECT TUBERCULOSIS?

Anecdotal evidence has linked tuberculosis to poverty-related environmental risk factors such as indoor air pollution, tobacco smoke, malnutrition, overcrowding, and excessive alcohol usage for decades. The most important defence against tuberculosis is a robust immune system where 60% of persons with a healthy immune system can totally kill TB bacteria. One of the familiar examples of environmental factors where tuberculosis is directly associated with HIV infected patients. One of the findings were reported where it showed some relationship between seasonal fluctuation in HIV-infected individuals with a pulmonary tuberculosis diagnosis (summer/autumn vs. winter/spring) and short-term exposure to environmental risk variables such temperature and ambient $NO_2$ and $SO_2$ (summer/autumn vs. winter/spring). These findings confirm the idea that seasonality and environmental variables have a role in predicting the incidence of pulmonary tuberculosis in HIV-positive people, and we hope that they will help guide future tuberculosis preventive studies throughout the world [18].

## CONCLUSION

In short, tuberculosis infection and illness are still common and observed in those populations where people live in poverty. Most of the cases related to tuberculosis are reported in overcrowded places where people live and work in poor ventilated area. So, these are the ideal conditions for any disease e.g. tuberculosis to grow and spread from one person to another. So, we will require a large medical facility with community-based organisations is an efficient way of providing highly targeted screening services to a population that is at high risk of disease acquisition and transmission. Most importantly, tuberculosis can also be avoided by limiting exposure to air pollution and other potentially harmful environmental factors. Another major cause of lung disease is air pollution, which must be addressed.

## REFERENCES

1. Tremblay, G.A. Historical Statistics Support a Hypothesis linking Tuberculosis and Air Pollution caused by coal. Int J Tuberc Lung Dis. 2007; 11: 722-732.
2. Lin, H.H., Ezzati, M. and Murray, M. Tobacco Smoke, Indoor Air Pollution and Tuberculosis: A Systematic review and meta-analysis. PLoS Med 2007; 4: e20.
3. Van Zyl Smit, R.N., Pai, M., Yew, W.W., *et al.* Global Lung Health: The Colliding Epidemics of Tuberculosis, Tobacco Smoking, HIV and COPD. Eur Respir J. 2010; 35: 27-33.
4. Weiss, M.G., Sommerfeld, J. and Uplekar, M.W. Social and Cultural Dimensions of Gender and Tuberculosis. Int J Tuberc Lung Dis. 2008; 12: 829-830.
5. Hwang, S., Kang, S., Lee, J.Y., Lee, J.S., Kim, H.J., Han, S.K., *et al.* Impact of Outdoor Air Pollution on the Incidence of Tuberculosis in the Seoul Metropolitan Area, South Korea. Korean J Intern Med. 2014; 29(2): 183-90.
6. Popovic, I., Magalhaes, R.J.S., Ge, E., Marks, G.B., Dong, G.H., Wei, X., *et al.* A Systematic Literature review and Critical Appraisal of Epidemiological Studies on Outdoor Air Pollution and Tuberculosis Outcomes. Environ Res. 2019; 170: 33-45.
7. Song, Q., Christiani, D.C., Xiaorong, W. and Ren, J. The Global Contribution of Outdoor Air Pollution to the Incidence, Prevalence, Mortality and Hospital Admission for Chronic Obstructive Pulmonary Disease: A Systematic review and meta-analysis. Int J Environ Res Public Health 2014;11(11): 11822-32.
8. Shah, I.M., Laaberki, M.H., Popham, D.L. and Dworkin, J. A Eukaryotic-like Ser/Thr kinase Signals Bacteria to exit Dormancy in Response to Peptidoglycan Fragments. Cell 2008; 135: 486-496.
9. Cambi, A., Koopman, M. and Figdor, C.G. How C-type Lectins detect Pathogens. Cell Microbiol 2005; 7: 481-488.
10. Cardona, P.J. A Dynamic Reinfection Hypothesis of Latent Tuberculosis Infection. Infection. 2009; 37: 80-86.
11. Yew, W.W. and Leung, C.C. Update in Tuberculosis 2007. Am J Respir Crit Care Med. 2008; 177: 479-485.
12. Amigorena, S., Drake, J.R., Webster, P. and Mellman, I. Transient Accumulation of New Class II MHC Molecules in a Novel Endocytic Compartment in B lymphocytes. Nature. 1994; 369: 113-120.
13. Kurmi, O.P., Sadhra, C.S., Ayres, J.G. and Sadhra, S.S. Tuberculosis Risk from exposure to Solid Fuel Smoke: A Systematic Review and Meta-analysis. J Epidemiol Community Health. 2014; 68(12): 1112-8.
14. Kolappan, C. and Subramani, R. Association between Biomass Fuel and Pulmonary Tuberculosis: A Nested Case–control Study. Thorax 2009; 64(8): 705-8.
15. Mehta, P.K., Raj, A., Singh, N. and Khuller, G.K. Diagnosis of Extrapulmonary Tuberculosis by PCR. FEMS Immunol Med Microbiol 2012; 66: 20-36.
16. Mendelson, M. Diagnosing Tuberculosis in HIV-infected Patients: Challenges and Future Prospects. Br Med Bull 2007; 81-82:149-165.

17. Ellis, R.D., Hatherill, M., Tait, D., Snowden, M., Churchyard, G., Hanekom, W. *et al.* Innovative Clinical Trial Designs to rationalize TB Vaccine Development. Tuberculosis 2015; 95: 352-357.

18. Jam, S., Sabzvari, D., Seyed Alinaghi, S., Fattahi, F., Jabbari, H. and Mohraz, M. Frequency of Mycobacterium Tuberculosis Infection among Iranian Patients with HIV/AIDS by PPD test. Acta Med Iran 2010; 48( 1): 67-71.

**Corresponding author: Dr Amit Gupta, Associate Professor, Department of Biotechnology, Graphic Era (Deemed to be) University, Dehradun, India.**
**Email id: dr.amitgupta.bt@geu.ac.in**

Pages: 48-54
Emerging Environmental Contaminants and Global Healthcare Systems
*Editors:* Prof. (Dr.) Shyam Narain Pandey; Murtaza Abid
Prof. (Dr.) Syed Rais Haider; Dr. Sabiha Kazmi; Dr. Mohd. Zahid Rizvi
*ISBN:* 978-81-959169-2-4
*Edition:* 2023
*Published by:* Discovery Publishing House, New Delhi (India)

# Environment Toxicants
## *Types, Sources and Effects*

**Khushi Kashyap and Amit Gupta**

### ABSTRACT

*Any harmful material created by humans or introduced into the environment as a result of human action is considered an environmental toxicant. As a result, toxicants cover a broad range of molecules, from inorganic elements like metals to a wide range of organic compounds like pharmaceutical medications. Environmental toxicants are any chemical or physical agents that can pollute the abiotic components of ecosystems, such as water, land, and air, impacting the environment in general and having poor health effects in biotic populations, such as animals, plants, and microbes. Toxicants exist in a variety of shapes and sizes, and while they can come from both natural and human-made sources, this course will focus on the consequences of human and environmental toxicants.*

***Keywords:*** *Environment; toxicants; human and natural.*

### INTRODUCTION

Toxicants can enter the human body by inhalation, skin contact, food, or water consumption. The presence of arsenic (As) in drinking water or lead (Pb) in the environment, for example, has become a major public health concern all over the world. Pesticides are equally dangerous to the environment and human health. Pesticides have contaminated drinking water supplies, vegetables, animal feed, milk, and seafood as a result of

Department of Biotechnology, Graphic Era (Deemed to be) University, Dehradun, (India)

their widespread use in agriculture. Pesticides, like heavy metals, have been linked to a slew of health problems [1]. In addition, certain chemical toxicants in our environment, such as pharmaceutical or chemical industry waste, act as endocrine disrupting agents and have been related to a variety of human disorders [1, 2].

## TYPES OF ENVIRONMENT TOXICANTS

The environment, as previously indicated, comprises a wide range of toxicants. To better understand them, we may classify them into categories based on the types of issues they cause, such as mutagens, teratogens, allergens, carcinogens, neurotoxins, and endocrine disrupters [3-6].

- *Mutagens:* Mutagen refers to anything that causes a change in sequence i.e. mutation. So, these mutagens may produce DNA alterations that can harm cells and cause several diseases like cancer. In addition, radioactive substances, X-rays, UV light, and some compounds are examples of mutagens.
- *Teratogens:* When a teratogen is introduced to a growing embryo or foetus, birth malformations or abnormalities may occur. During development in the womb, these substances may cause birth abnormalities. Thalidomide was used as a sleeping drug and to ease nausea during pregnancy in the 1950s, but it was later discovered to be a very harmful teratogen. A single intake of the substance has the potential to induce serious birth abnormalities in offspring.
- *Allergens:* An allergy respond only when a person reacts to elements in the environment that are ordinarily benign to most people. Dust mites, pets, pollen, insects, parasites, moulds, foods, and some medicines are all sources of allergens.
- *Carcinogens:* Carcinogens are substances or situations that have the potential to cause cancer. Tobacco, chemicals in the environment, medical radiation, and even infections and drugs are all examples. Carcinogens, or cancer-causing substances, are arguably the most well-known toxicants.
- *Neurotoxins:* Neurotoxins are poisonous or harmful to nerve tissue, causing damage to the organism's central nervous system. Pesticides and chemical weapons, as well as heavy metals like lead and mercury, are among them. Neurotoxins can cause slurred speech, a loss of muscle function, and even death.
- *Endocrine disruptors:* Chemicals that mimic or interfere with the body's hormones, which are controlled by the endocrine system, are known as endocrine disruptors. The hormone system, commonly known as the endocrine system, is responsible for regulating growth, development, sexual maturity, cognitive function, and even appetite.

## SOURCES OF ENVIRONMENT TOXICANTS

Toxicants can arise from a variety of places, but they tend to flow through the environment in predictable patterns. Toxicants can be transported by runoff from wide areas of land and end up in aquatic systems. Toxicants tend to concentrate in the water because water systems are smaller than the area where the toxins were formed. There are a variety of environmental toxins that might get up in our food sources including water, or air. Other major sources include chemical and inorganic pollutants including pesticides, and biological agents, all of which can harm living beings. We are surrounded by synthetic chemicals and come into contact with them on a regular basis. Plastics, household cleaners, detergents, cosmetics, and perfumes are all toxicants. Antibiotics, prescription drugs, steroids, food additives, preservatives, and other things that we ingest all have the potential to be dangerous. Pesticides, herbicides, and fertilisers are examples of toxicants [7-10].

- ***Plastics:*** Long-term use and high-temperature exposure of plastics and plastic items can cause harmful chemical elements to leak into food, drinks, and water. Harmful substances can be emitted into the air as a result of indiscriminate land dumping of plastics and open-air burning, constituting a public health danger. As a result of indiscriminate land dumping of plastics and open-air burning, harmful compounds can be released into the air, posing a public health risk.
- ***Home cleansers:*** Many cleaning products and household items can irritate the eyes and throat, as well as cause headaches and other health problems like cancer. Hazardous substances, such as volatile organic compounds (VOCs), are emitted by some goods (VOCs). Two more potentially harmful compounds are ammonia and bleach.
- ***Detergents:*** Our bodies are exposed to 1,4-Dioxane and other hazardous substances found in detergents. These chemicals not only stay in clothes after they've been washed, but they can also go into your skin if your clothes get damp or wet.
- ***Cosmetics:*** Cosmetics have a bad environmental impact, regardless of whether the product or by-product is washed down or drain into the sink or thrown away in the garbage. In contrast, chemicals and toxins released from industries may directly effect and pollute our earth and water bodies and also showed its deleterious effect on wildlife habitat, and more.
  - In landfills, cosmetic packaging can take hundreds of years to disintegrate, releasing chemicals into the soil and waterways in the process.
  - Most conventional cosmetics include toxic substances, which eventually find their way into our land and oceans, harming natural environment and wildlife.

- Pesticides used on raw ingredients during farming harm the environment because they infiltrate into the soil and end up in bodies of water.
- Palm oil is used in a variety of products and is a major contributor to deforestation, species loss, and climate change.
- Turtles and marine animals absorb micro beads, wet wipes, and plastic packaging, which block their digestive tracts and kill them.
- The toxic ingredients found in popular sunscreens are decimating corals and marine eco systems at an alarming rate.

• ***Perfumes:*** A volatile chemical ingredient is present in each spritz of perfume. According to NOAA, once sprayed, VOCs react with sunshine and other substances in the atmosphere to generate ozone pollution.

## EFFECTS OF ENVIRONMENT TOXICANTS ON HUMANS

Endocrine disrupting chemicals (EDCs), also referred as hormone disrupting compounds, are prevalent in the environment. Hormone-producing glands in our endocrine system include the thyroid and pituitary glands, for example. These hormones assist in the control of body functions. Toxins are chemical molecules created by humans that interfere with the regular functioning of our hormones.

EDCs disturb the hormonal process at any point along the way, from the gland that makes the hormone to the tissue that absorbs it, and everywhere in between. We still have a lot to learn about how the disruption happens, but we do know that it does. EDCs have been related to cancer, heart disease, and reproductive issues in studies [11-13].

• Pregnancy, obesity, diabetes, and heart disease are all affected by EDCs.
• Impact of EDC on:
  - ***Pregnancy:*** Menopause begins earlier, sperm quality deteriorates, and fertility issues arise.
  - ***Obesity:*** Exposure to BPA (e.g. industrial chemical used in plastics), phthalates (e.g. usage in plastics), arsenic, and several other EDCs has been shown to impact metabolic illnesses in cellular and animal models (such as diabetes and obesity).
  - ***Diabetes:*** DDE, a chemical, has been linked to diabetes. DDE is formed when the body breaks down DDT (a pesticide that was banned in 1972 but is still found in nature), as well as EDC levels and obesity.
  - ***Heart Disease:*** EDCs have been established in animal models to have a deleterious influence on cardiovascular health.

## LIBERAL LIMITATIONS ON DANGEROUS SUBSTANCES IN THE ENVIRONMENT POSE A SIGNIFICANT CHALLENGE TO ENVIRONMENTAL TOXICITY

- There are no hard and fast rules when it comes to some health risks. Human doses of radioactivity have been calculated based on natural type of exposure due to radiation from the Earth (e.g. Radon and Uranium) as well as ionising radiation from outer space.
- Humans are frequently affected by high-dose radiation of more than 150 mSv. Due to the direct exposure of specific radiation at a very low level may cause some change in the cellular DNA and showed several abnormalities.
- The higher the dose of radiation, the greater the risk of DNA abnormalities and mutations, which can lead to cancer [14].
- As a result, reducing exposure reduces the health risk; nevertheless, there is no hard and fast rule; even a single impact can damage DNA.
- When defining pollution guidelines, other environmental factors must be taken into account. Organic molecules, in example, can change when exposed to intense UV radiation or when pH in water changes.
- In various ways, these things may or may not be harmful. Things become much more complicated when several contaminants are mixed together.
- During screening analysis of ground, drinking, or waste water, it is impossible to screen for thousands of potentially dangerous compounds, thus the laboratory work soon outweighs the cost limits. For Example: 2, 3, 7, 8-tetrachlorodibenzo-p-dioxin (2, 3, 7, 8-TCDD), also known as dioxin, had never been manufactured for commercial use and had only been used as a research test chemical. As a result, no routine testing was done until it caused the Seveso poisoning in Italy [15].

## SYNOPSIS OF A CASE STUDY

The effects of short-lived radon derivatives at levels close to the current occupational limit on lung cancer mortality were studied in 1415 Swedish iron workers. Lung cancer claimed the lives of 50 persons between 1951 and 1976, compared to 12.8 anticipated.

## AWARENESS

People being more aware of toxicants from anthropogenic sources helps to maintain the ecological balance of the system by lowering toxicant input rates. All conceivable steady states of the system are given existence and local asymptotic stability requirements. When there are very high levels of contaminants in the system, zooplankton vanishes. Importantly, the restricted quantity of extra food for zooplankton keeps the aquatic food web system from collapsing. The findings suggest that environmental pollutants can be controlled to a low level by raising human consciousness, hence sustaining the planktonic ecosystem's rhythm.

## CONCLUSION

Toxins in the environment can be identified and avoided; to be honest, entirely avoiding them is unrealistic. Many companies are making an attempt to avoid using chemicals. When consumers want more natural products from conscientious producers, this trend will continue. So, frontiers in Environmental Toxicity is envisioned as a novel platform for monitoring environmental safety levels and also detecting or preventing accidental releases of harmful substances into the environment alone or in combination with other pollutants and directly affect our biotic and abiotic factors.

## REFERENCES


1. Albretsen, J. The Toxicity of Iron, an Essential Element; Veterinary Medicine 2006; 82-90.
2. Andia, J.B. Aluminium Toxicity: Its Relationship with Bone and Iron Metabolism. Nephrol Dial Transplant 1996; 11(Suppl 3): 69-73.
3. Flora, S.J.S., Mittal, M. and Mehta, A. Heavy Metal Induced Oxidative Stress & its possible Reversal by Chelation Therapy. Indian J Med Res 2008; 128: 501-523.
4. Han, J.X., Shang, Q. and Du, Y. Effect of Environmental Cadmium Pollution on Human Health. Health 2009; 1(3): 159-166.
5. Khlifi, R. and Hamza-Chaffai, A. Head and Neck Cancer due to Heavy Metal exposure via Tobacco Smoking and Professional exposure: A Review. Toxicol Appl Pharmacol 2010; 248: 71-88.
6. Kochian, L.V., Piñeros, M.A. and Hoekenga, O.A. The Physiology, Genetics and Molecular Biology of Plant Aluminum Resistance and Toxicity. Plant and Soil 2005; 274: 175-195.
7. Martin S, Griswold W. Human Health Effects of Heavy Metals. Environmental Science and Technology Briefs for Citizens 2009; (15): 1-6.
8. Villanueva C, Kogevinas M, Cordier S, Templeton M, Vermeulen R, Nuckols J. Assessing exposure and Health Consequences of Chemicals in Drinking Water: Current State of knowledge and Research needs. Environ. Health Perspect 2013; 122: 213-221.
9. Vogt R, Bennett D, Cassady D, Frost J, Ritz B, Hertz-Picciotto I. Cancer and Non-cancer Health effects from Food Contaminant exposures for Children and Adults in California: A Risk Assessment. Environ. Health 2012; 11: 83.
10. Shen R, Andrews S. Demonstration of 20 Pharmaceuticals and Personal Care Products (PPCPs) as Nitrosamine Precursors during Chloramine Disinfection. Water Res 2011; 45, 944-952.
11. Axelstad M. *et al.* EDC IMPACT: Reduced Sperm Counts in Rats exposed to Human Relevant mixtures of Endocrine Disrupters. Endocr Connect 2018; 7: 139-148.
12. Skakkebaek NE. A brief Review of the Link between Environment and Male Reproductive Health: Lessons from Studies of Testicular Germ Cell Cancer. Horm Res Paediatr 2016; 86: 240-246.

13. Heindel JJ, Skalla LA, Joubert BR, Dilworth CH, Gray KA. Review of Developmental Origins of Health and Disease Publications in Environmental Epidemiology. Reprod Toxicol 2017; 68: 34-48.
14. Azzam, EI, de Toledo SM, Gooding T, Little JB. Intercellular Communication is involved in the bystander Regulation of Gene Expression in Human Cells exposed to very Low Fluences of Alpha Particles. Radiat Res 1998; 150: 497-504.
15. Barcellos-Hoff MH, Park C, Wright EG. Radiation and the Microenvironment—tumorigenesis and Therapy. Nat Rev Cancer 2005; 5: 867-875.

**Corresponding author: Dr Amit Gupta, Associate Professor, Department of Biotechnology, Graphic Era (Deemed to be) University, Dehradun, India.**
**Email id: dr.amitgupta.bt@geu.ac.in**

Pages: 55-64
**Emerging Environmental Contaminants and Global Healthcare Systems**
*Editors:* **Prof. (Dr.) Shyam Narain Pandey; Murtaza Abid**
**Prof. (Dr.) Syed Rais Haider; Dr. Sabiha Kazmi; Dr. Mohd. Zahid Rizvi**
*ISBN:* **978-81-959169-2-4**
*Edition:* **2023**
*Published by:* **Discovery Publishing House, New Delhi (India)**

# Green Nanotechnology and Environment

**Vidhi Pansuriya, *Harmanpreet Kaur, *Amit Gupta**

## ABSTRACT

*According to the technology advancement in the field of environment is one of the major challenges. Whenever, engineers had tried to elevate world with their inventions, environmental health comes into trouble. Be it invention of automobile or plastic bags, humans have always suffocated nature to pace up the game of development. Resolution of one problem has led to a new problem. To combat issues related to environment, a novel technique of green nanotechnology was proposed. Post the success of nanotechnology in various fields, researchers decided to apply nanotechnology to sustain the environment and its resources. Nanotechnology deals with the field of science which designs and function on nanoscale. Nanotechnology, a transdisciplinary breakthrough technology that is used to develop creative solutions in the industries (i.e. primary/secondary/tertiary/quaternary), has made modest development due to the possible concerns of nanotoxicity. To counter this, green and eco-friendly nanotechnology solutions play a key role in achieving sustainable development goals and removing the risk of technification of innovation process. In this article, a depth study of green nanotechnology shall be discussed.*

***Keywords:*** *sustainable development, nanotechnology, nanoscale and green nanotechnology.*

## INTRODUCTION

Nanotechnology has a wide range of applications, from classic chemical processes to medical and environmental technologies. Nanotechnology is

**Infinity Pathology Laboratory, Katargam, Surat, Gujarat**
***Department of Biotechnology, Graphic Era (Deemed to be) University, Dehradun, (India)**

considered as a vital technology of the twenty-first century and has produced a lot of enthusiasm throughout the world, but it has been held down due to a lack of knowledge of the hazards related with nanotechnology and a lack of rules to control new risks. Researchers, on the other hand, continue to go ahead, committing to overcoming hurdles ranging from managing, producing, funding, regulatory, and technological elements. Green nanotechnology is a subset of green technology that employs principles from green chemistry and green engineering, with the term "green" referring to the utilisation of plant products. It saves energy and gasoline by utilising less material and renewable inputs whenever possible. Furthermore, nanotechnological goods, processes, and applications are predicted to considerably contribute to environmental and climate protection by conserving raw materials, energy, and water, as well as lowering greenhouse gas emissions and hazardous waste [1, 2]. Green nanotechnology's key advantages include increased energy efficiency, reduced waste and greenhouse gas emissions, and reduced use of non-renewable raw resources. Green nanotechnology provides an excellent chance to avert negative consequences before they arise. Green nanotechnology should be introduced (Figure 8.1) and considered as one of the efficient and more effective replacement compared with synthetic nanotechnology, hereby to introduce and addressing some environmental challenges which incorporates basic principle related to green science.

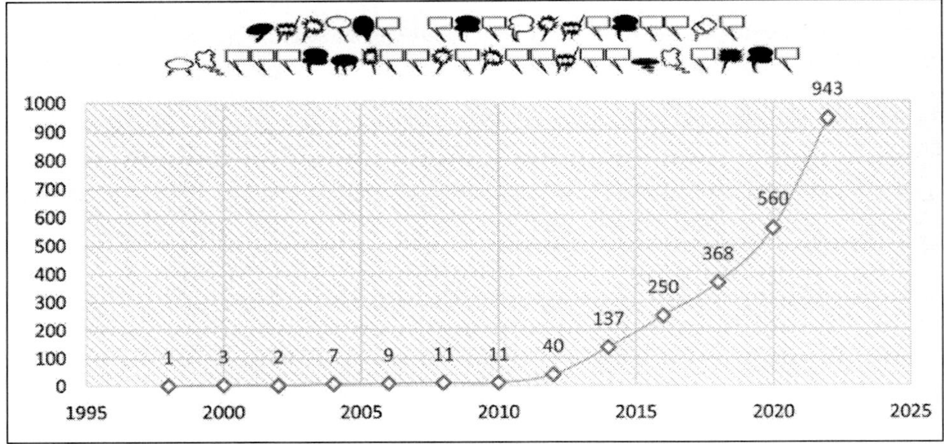


**Fig. 8.1**

Some of the most familiar examples related to green science e.g. nanomaterials production and its coproducts without harming or damaging the environment or human health, using the least amount of energy possible, and also used less amount of waste/pollution possible. In this regard, approaches and processes were applied related to nanotechnology i.e. solid-state reactions, conservation of energy, usage of water sources instead of organic solvents. These approaches and processes mainly modifying the structure of nanomaterials to reduce toxicity, and variables related to recyclability and reusability are critical.

### Preface to Understand Green Nanotechnology

Green nanotechnology is the applied part of nanotechnology that was introduced to develop such technologies that not only sustain human health but our environment too. It works towards elevating the sustainability in technologies associated with environmental development [3]. It basically involves manufacturing of green nanoparticles or green products, which are the two goals that green nanotechnology aims at for maintenance of sustainability. Some prime pointers to be kept in conscience while manufacturing green nanoparticles or green products are:

- No use of toxic ingredients.
- Usage of less energy at lower temperatures
- As far as possible use renewable inputs
- Making roadmaps

Green nanotechnology uses principles of green engineering as its baseline [4]. A list of twelve principles is given as under:

- Prevent waste
- Atom economy
- Less hazardous chemical synthesis
- Designing safer chemicals
- Safer solvents or reaction media
- Design for energy efficiency
- Renewable feedstock
- Reduce derivatives
- Catalysis
- Degradation design
- Real time monitoring and process control
- Inherently safer chemicals

A brief about its application and practice is given in the diagram given below (Figure 8.2).

## TYPES OF GREEN NANOPARTICLES

The availability of plant chemical groups with substantial physiochemical capabilities facilitates the use of plants to combine nature and science. Aside from the safety of plant-derived nanoparticles, nanostructures are non-toxic to environment [5]. The size, surface properties, and targeting moieties of nanostructures all contribute to these advantages.

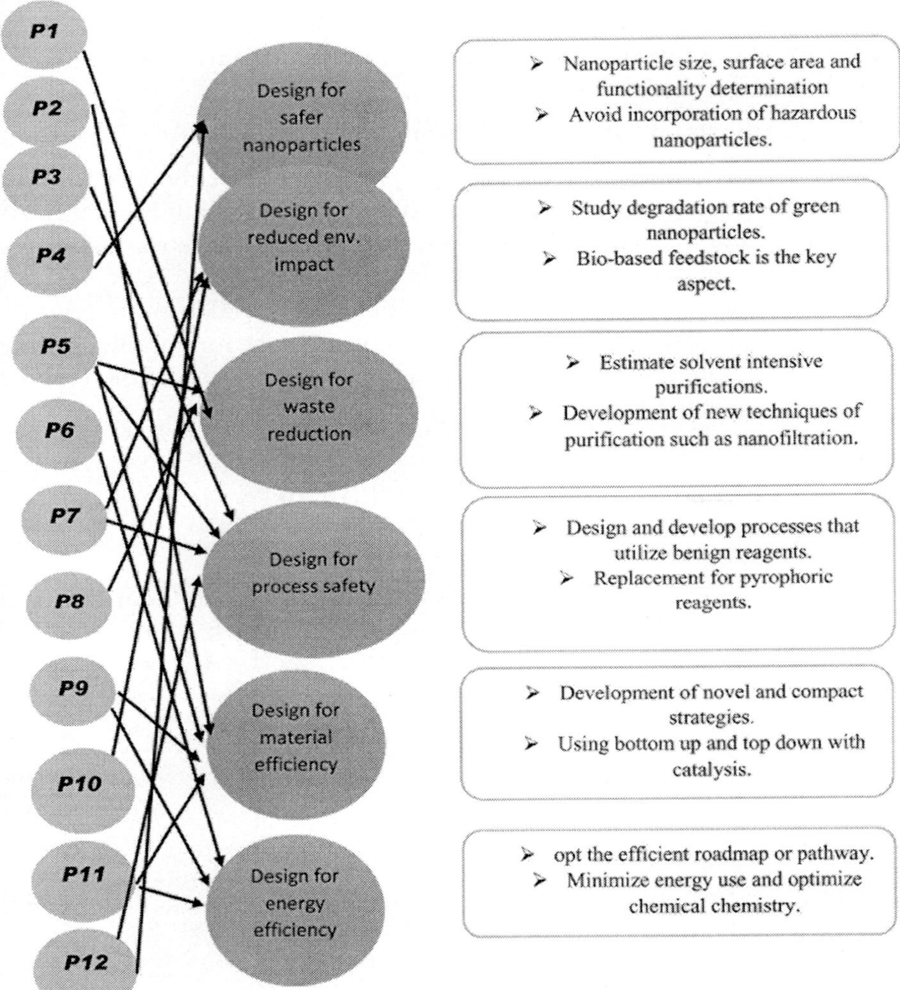


**Fig. 8.2: Application and practices of Nanotechnology**

These amazing properties of green nanostructures let to the discovery of nanodrugs also. Several studies have been published on the use of phytochemicals and plant extracts as reducing and stabilising agents in the green production of metal and metal oxide nanoparticles.

Phenolic based nanoparticles are secondary metabolites that defend plants from insects, fungus, bacteria, and viruses. They are the most diverse group of phytochemicals, with about 7900 compounds discovered in various plant sources. As significant phenolics, flavonoids are among the most important and varied secondary metabolites discovered in many plants.

In reality, they are a vast class of polyphenolics made up of a basic flavonoid's nucleus coupled by a three-carbon atom heterocyclic ring to two aromatic rings [6,7]. Table 8.1 given below represents the metal nanoparticles derived from plants:

**Table 8.1: Plants used for synthesizing nanoparticles**

| Nanoparticles | Plant Used |
|---|---|
| Au | |
| • | *llium sativum* |
| • | *Azadirachta indica A. Juss* |
| • | *Benincasa hispida* |
| • | *Camellia sinensis* |
| • | *Justicia gendarussa* |
| • | *Magnolia Kobus* |
| • | *Mirabilis jalapa* |
| • | *Saraca indica* |
| • | *Syzygium aromaticum* |
| • | *Terminalia catappa* |
| Cu/CuO | |
| • | *Aloe barbadensis* |
| • | *Calotropis procera L.* |
| • | *Euphorbia nivulia* |
| • | *Terminalia arjuna* |
| • | *Tridax procumbens* |
| Ag | |
| • | *Trianthema decandra* |
| • | *Terminalia chebula* |
| • | *Solanum xanthocarpum* |
| • | *Plumeria rubra* |
| • | *Piper nigrum* |
| • | *Piper betle* |
| • | *Phoma glomerata* |
| • | *Pinus eldarica* |
| • | *Pelargonium graveolens* |
| • | *Pedilanthus tithymaloides* |
| • | *Parthenium hysterophorus* |
| • | *Ocimum tenuiflorum* |
| • | *Morinda pubescens* |
| • | *Leonuri herba* |
| • | *Lantana camara* |
| • | *Hydrilla verticilata* |

*(Table Contd...)*

| | |
|---|---|
| • <br>• <br>• <br>• <br>• <br>• <br>• <br>• <br>• <br>• <br>• <br>• <br>• <br>• <br>• | *Hydrilla sp.*<br>*Hibiscus cannabinus*<br>*Glycyrrhiza Glabra*<br>*Festuca rubra*<br>*Eucalyptus hybrida*<br>*Elettaria cardamomom*<br>*Dioscorea oppositifolia*<br>*Dioscorea bulbifera*<br>*Desmodium triflorum*<br>*Delonix elata*<br>*Datura metel*<br>*Alternanthera sessilis Linn*<br>*Andrographis paniculata Nees*<br>*Astragalus gummifer Labill*<br>*Azadirachta indica* |
| pd<br>• <br>• <br>• <br>• <br>• | <br>*Annona squamosa*<br>*Cinnamomum zeylanicum*<br>*Gardenia jasminoides Ellis*<br>*Glycine max*<br>*Piper betle* |

## PRODUCTION OF NEXT GENERATION NANOMATERIALS

The process of producing plant-based nanomaterials is termed as 'green synthesis of nanomaterials (Figure 8.3). Manufacturing process of green nanomaterials involves three processes namely:

- *Selection of plant extract:* It is the initial step in green synthesis where selection of plant extract possessing potential properties of biological reduction of metallic ions and hyper-accumulation for the process to be taken forward. In general, plant extracts having bioactive molecules (i.e. alkaloids, flavonoids, phenolic acids, terpenoids, and polyphenols) which played a vital or effective role pertaining stabilising metallic ions [8]. Determination of active biomolecules in terms of its concentration and content which may be helpful in finding out the size and form of nanoparticles.
- *Selection of ionic source:* Aqueous mellitic ions are most preferred ion source for this process. Metal salt precursors (i.e. aqueous ion) may be helpful and more effective in order to decline in nanoparticles synthesis. So, this may due to change in colour reaction mixture and marked as one of the indicator (quantitative) of nanoparticle generation. In general, nanoparticles produced from reducing agents may be harmful or toxic so we need to focus and more concern about

ecologically acceptable methods. So, nanoparticles production is mainly produced through mixing of plant extract with metal ion solution. Firstly, reduction in biochemical content in the salt solution which may responsible for synthesizing nanoparticles. For confirmation of its synthesis, we observe colour change in the reaction mixture. In contrast, activation step of nanoparticles synthesis, metal ions are changed to zero-valent states i.e. monovalent or divalent oxidation states, allowing for the nucleation of such reduced metal atoms.

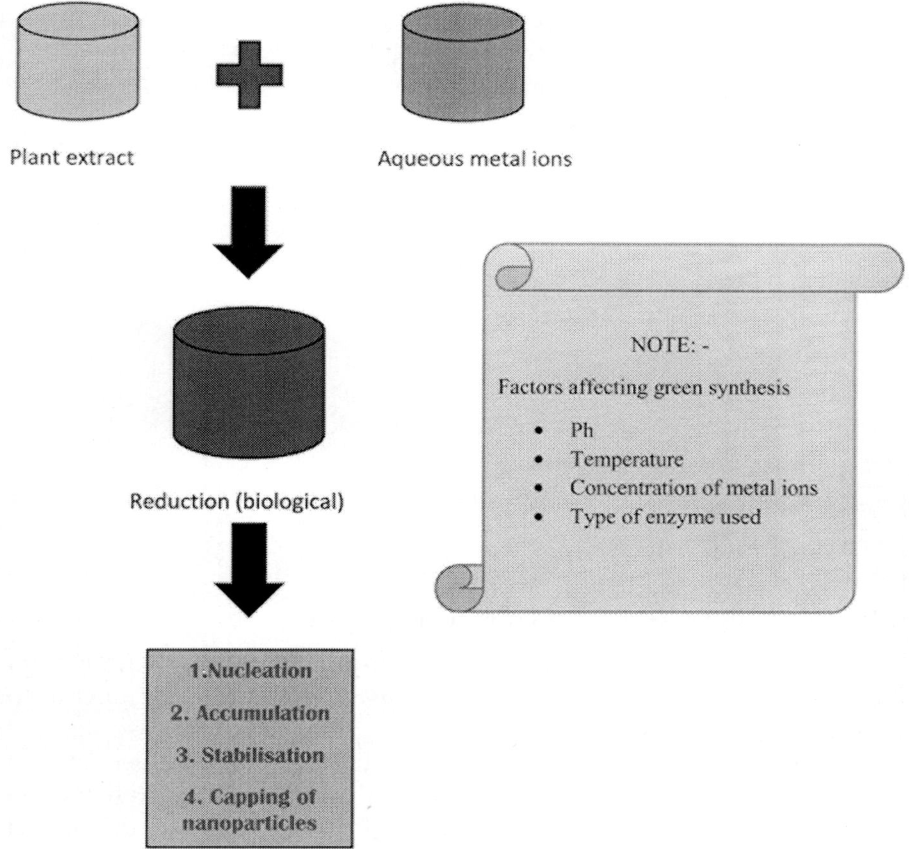


**Fig. 8.3: Green synthesis of metal nanoparticles**

- *Integration of particles:* The process of nanoparticle formation is followed by the integration of smaller neighbouring particles to produce bigger thermodynamically stable nanoparticles, and the metal ions are then reduced biologically. As a result, growth continues and nanoparticles consolidate to form spheres, cubes, triangles, rods, wires, hexagons, and pentagons [9]. The capacity of plant extract to stabilise the nanoparticle influences its stable shape in the final step of the procedure. The concentration, reaction duration, metal salt concentration, reaction solution pH, and temperature of the plant extracts all have a significant impact on the quality, size, and shape of the nanoparticles.

## GREEN NANOTECHNOLOGY AND GLOBAL ENVIRONMENTAL GOALS

Nanotechnology (NT) and Information, Communication, and Computation Technologies (ICCT) are referred to as 21st century technologies, and they have the potential to help achieve the United Nations' Sustainable Development Goals, which set a target of protecting the planet and ensuring peace and prosperity by 2030. To balance social, economic, and environmental sustainability, SD objectives and appropriate 21st-century technology are needed [10-12]. To achieve each SD target based on the issue's maximum or minimal goal. Appropriate technologies are chosen and presented. Nanotechnology and ICCT, independently or in combination, are said to be capable of achieving global sustainable objectives to a greater extent within the 15-year deadline. Some among those goals are listed below:

1. Clean water and sanitation
2. Affordable renewable energy
3.. Sustainable industrialization
4. Ensure sustainable Production & Consumption
5. Combat on Climate Change
6. Conserve Ocean & Marine Resources
7. Protect life on Land
8. Global Partnership for Sustainability

## APPLICATIONS OF GREEN NANOTECHNOLOGY

Green Technology (GT) is an environmental healing technology that lowers the environmental damage caused by items and technologies designed for people's convenience. GT is thought to increase agricultural income while decreasing environmental deterioration and conserving natural resources [13]. Green technologies are those that are environmentally friendly and do not leave a carbon footprint when applied in a variety of processes and applications. Green technologies promote the utilisation of natural organic resources while reducing the generation of greenhouse gases. They also use fewer resources and do not contribute to the universe's entropy. Green technology does not promote environmental damage [14, 15]. It has its some of major applications in agriculture, pharmaceutical, biochemical, automobile, IT sectors etc.

- Green nanotechnology is primarily used in agriculture sector to minimise environmental damage in agricultural operations aided by nanotechnology, particularly insect control.

- In food processing sector green synthesis is used to remove harmful elements in food and to minimise green gas emissions and environmental deterioration in all food packaging processes using green nanotechnology.
- It aims to develop environmentally friendly nanotechnological techniques for gathering potential natural energy sources in order to meet human civilization's energy needs without harming the environment.
- To manufacture energy-efficient, zero-emissions, long-lasting autos with renewable energy techniques based on green nanotechnology.
- Green nanotechnology and green techniques are used in all health and medical services. Nanotechnology synthesised plant-based drugs are widely used in oncology.
- In aero craft engineering, green energy and green nanomaterials, as well as ecologically acceptable nanotechnological techniques, are being used commercially.

## REFERENCES

1. Smith S, Geoff B. (2012). Green Nanophotonics. Journal of Nanophotonics 6(1): 061505.
2. Aithal B, Shubhra J, Aithal PS. (2020). Green and Eco-friendly Nanotechnology – Concepts and Industrial Prospects. International Journal of Management Technology and Social Sciences 6(1): 1-31.
3. Kuppusamy P, Yusoff MM, Maniam GP, Govindan N. (2016). Biosynthesis of Metallic Nanoparticles using Plant Derivatives and their New Avenues in Pharmacological Applications—an updated report. Saudi Pharm J 24(4): 473-484.
4. Isaac R, Sakthivel G, Murthy C. (2013). Green Synthesis of Gold and Silver Nanoparticles using *Averrhoa bilimbi* Fruit extract. J Nanotechnology: 6.
5. Ahmad S, Munir S, Zeb N, Ullah A, Khan B, Ali J, Muhammad B, Omer M, Alamzeb M, Syed SM, Ali S. (2019). Green Nanotechnology: A Review on Green Synthesis of Silver Nanoparticles — an Ecofriendly Approach. International Journal of Nanomedicine 14: 5087-5107.
6. Zou H, Wu S, Shen J. (2008). Polymer/silica Nanocomposites: Preparation, Characterization, Properties, and Applications. Chem Rev 108, 3893-3957.
7. Verma A, Gautam S, Bansal K, Prabhakar N, Rosenholm J (2019). Green Nanotechnology: Advancement in Phytoformulation Research. Medicines, 6(1), 39-44.
8. EPA Office of Research and Development. Draft Nanomaterial Research Strategy (NRS), January 24, 2008. U.S. Environmental Protection Agency Website. http://es.epa.gov/ncer/nano/publications/nano_strategy_012408.pdf (accessed February 2008).
9. Helland A, Wick P, Koehler A, Schmid K, Som C. (2007). Reviewing the Environmental and Human Health Knowledge Base of Carbon Nanotubes. Environ. Health Perspect 115, 1125-1131.
10. Schmidt, K.F. Green Nanotechnology: It's Easier Than You Think; Project on Emerging Nanotechnologies PEN 8; Woodrow Wilson International Center for Scholars: Washington, DC, April 2007. http://www.nanotechproject.org/file download/files/GreenNano_PEN8. Pdf.

11. Hutchison H, James E. (2008). Greener Nanoscience: A Proactive Approach to Advancing Applications and Reducing Implications of Nanotechnology. ACS Nano, 2(3), 395-402.
12. Dhingra R, Naidu S, Upreti, G, Sawhney R. (2010). Sustainable Nanotechnology: Through Green Methods and Life-Cycle Thinking. Sustainability 2(10): 3323-3338.
13. Badnjevic A. (2017). [IFMBE Proceedings] CMBEBIH 2017 Volume 62 | | Towards Green Nanotechnology: Maximizing benefits and Minimizing Harm, 10.1007/978-981-10-4166-2 (Chapter 26), 164-170.
14. Morganti P, Palombo M, Carezzi F, Nunziata M, Morganti G, Cardillo M, Chianese A. (2016). Green Nanotechnology serving the Bioeconomy: Natural Beauty Masks to Save the Environment. Cosmetics 3(4), 41-45.
15. Shamim N, Sharma VK. (2013). Sustainable Nanotechnology and the Environment: Advances and Achievements Volume 1124 | | Ten Years of Green Nanotechnology, 10.1021/bk-2013-1124, 1-10.

---

**Corresponding author: Dr Amit Gupta, Associate Professor, Department of Biotechnology, Graphic Era (Deemed to be) University, Dehradun, India.**
**Email id: dr.amitgupta.bt@geu.ac.in**

Pages: 65-74
**Emerging Environmental Contaminants and Global Healthcare Systems**
*Editors:* **Prof. (Dr.) Shyam Narain Pandey; Murtaza Abid**
**Prof. (Dr.) Syed Rais Haider; Dr. Sabiha Kazmi; Dr. Mohd. Zahid Rizvi**
*ISBN:* **978-81-959169-2-4**
*Edition:* **2023**
*Published by:* **Discovery Publishing House, New Delhi (India)**

# The Ocean Biome
## *Diverse Habitats and Marine Life*

**Smriti Khare, Saloni Gupta, Amit Gupta**

## ABSTRACT

*The ocean biome is populated with a diverse variety of organisms that live in the water and on the seafloor. Marine biology is the study of marine life and ecosystems. With underwater expeditions and submarine exploration, marine science brings people closer to the seafloor, so that that we can better understand these lifeforms and their contributions to the marine environment. The resources of the sea are vast, but their exploitation has significant consequences for our environment. Pollutants such as pesticides, fertilizers, and oil spills from tankers enter oceans, spreading along coastlines. These substances negatively affect marine life—and our way of life as well. Marine biologists need to work closely with manufacturers, designers, and other scientists to develop biotechnologies that are robust, cost-effective and sustainable for the marine environment.*

***Keywords:*** *Biome; ocean; marine; habitat and environment*

## INTRODUCTION

We live on a planet dominated by the ocean. Almost 71% of the earth's surface is covered by this vast region, which is the last great expanse to be explored and charted on this planet. Since the beginning of recorded history, scientists and naturalists have been fascinated with the diversity of marine organisms. This rich history has contributed greatly to our understanding of the modern world. Life in the oceans and brackish waters is studied in

**Department of Life Sciences and Biotechnology, Graphic Era Deemed to be University, Dehradun, (India)**

marine biology, which includes organisms such as corals that influence the shape of the seafloor. In marine biology, organisms such as archaea, bacteria, and marine mammals are examined. Additionally, ocean biology may be influenced by human activities, such as overfishing or fisheries [1, 2].

Ocean phenomena play a key role in controlling the distribution of organisms in marine biology. The understanding of food chains, predator-prey relationships, and marine ecosystem dynamics is a major focus of the study. It is crucial for the fisheries industry to obtain information on fish and crustacean populations in the marine environment. Marine biology also focuses on polluting the oceans with certain types of pollutants, such as pesticides and fertilizers drained from land sources, oil spills from tankers, and silt built up along coastlines. Biological and ecological models have proven invaluable for identifying and developing biotechnologies based on marine resources. New antifouling technologies and UV-absorbing materials are being developed as a result of this approach. In the near future, manufacturers will be forced to develop new technologies that are acceptable to the environment and health as currently produced products are phased out. Marine biology fundamental research linked with applications directly related to it plays a crucial role in discovering new and unique biotechnological advances [3].

## IMPORTANCE OF MARINE BIOLOGY

- **To conserve marine biodiversity and the terrestrial environment**

Approximately 80% of the life on earth lives in the oceans, and the sea has been home to life for about 3 billion years now. Thousands of phytoplankton and tens of thousands of zooplankton may be in a mouthful of seawater. In the world's oceans, three times as much garbage is dumped as fish are caught every year. Plastic pellets are six times more abundant than zooplankton in some areas of the North Pacific Ocean. Organisms ingesting plastic will be killed because it is not biodegradable. Biomagnification causes many industrial chemicals to biodegrade and kill top predators. Fish can develop sex changes or infertility when certain chemicals bind to their hormone receptors. Understanding these connections helps us develop more effective regulations.

Together, phytoplankton and algae are much more important to global photosynthesis than land plants due to their use of $CO_2$ dissolved in seawater. Therefore, marine photosynthetic organisms are capable of minimizing the amount of $CO_2$ dissolved in the oceans and therefore in the atmosphere, which has important implications for all life. In addition, many marine habitats are buffer zones that reduce the impact of storm surges and tsunamis on coastal areas. Coral reefs and mangroves are examples of such habitats [3, 4].

- **To preserve our fisheries and food source**

Humans consume about 70% of their protein from fish, yet fisheries are overfished and unsustainable. Biologists study fisheries pertaining to measured its maximum sustainable yield, or quantity of fish which is mainly harvested continuously from a stock under current environmental conditions, without interfering with the regeneration of the fishery [5, 6].

- **For medical purposes and human health**

Since coral has a similar architecture and chemical properties to human bone, it is utilized for bone grafting, assisting in the healing of bones. Research on regeneration often uses echinoderms and other invertebrates. Invertebrates especially sponges contain several chemicals that are used to produce a wide variety of pharmaceuticals. The marine environment produces new compounds regularly. Shellfish poisoning or ciguatera can be caused by certain phytoplankton species. To control outbreaks and reduce human health risks, biologists need an understanding of these species' biology [4-6].

## MARINE HABITAT

Habitats are ecological or environmental zones that support individual species of animals, plants, or other organisms. From the tiny layers of surface water between ocean and atmosphere, where organisms may be trapped by the surface tension, to the depths of the oceanic trenches, sometimes 10,000 meters below the surface of the ocean, Marine Biology studies a wide range of habitats. There are three general types of marine habitat [7, 8], which are:

- **The Benthic zone:** In an ocean, a lake or a sea, there is a region below the surface of sediments and beneath some layers below the sediment surface called the Benthic zone.
- **The Demersal zone:** This definition refers to the part of the sea or ocean comprising the water column located close to the seabed and benthos (and consequently influenced by them). Unlike the benthos, which comes before the demersal zone, the demersal zone is above the seabed. Seafloors and the life that lives there can have a significant impact on it.
- **The Pelagic zone:** An open sea or ocean is classified as a pelagic zone if it lies away from the coast or seafloor. From the surface of the sea all the way down to the bottom, the pelagic zone consists of an imaginary cylinder of water.

## MARINE BIODIVERSITY

A species' level of complexity, as well as the variation between ecosystems, is what we mean by marine biodiversity [9-11].

- **Marine Micro-organisms:** Oceans are dominated by micro-organisms. In addition to viruses, bacteria and cyanobacteria, archaea and protozoa, they include stromatolites, haptophytes, alveolates, choanoflagellates and amoeboid protozoa. The barely visible insects play important ecological roles, even though they can't be seen by the naked eye. Their role in decomposition and nutrient recycling is key to the functioning of food chains
- **Marine Primary Producers:** Phytoplankton, which is a small but extremely abundant group of photosynthetic micro-organisms that live in the water column, provides most of the ocean's primary production. The multicellular primary producers, such as seaweeds (the red algae, green algae, and brown algae) and flowering plants, can only grow in shallow coastal areas because they require attachment to the benthos. They contribute to the detrital food chain, provide habitat for many animals, and contribute to primary production in these ecosystems. Additionally, they trap and stabilize sediment through their roots.
- In the marine environment, seagrasses are the best-adapted flowering plants, as they live underwater. Both tropical and temperate waters are home to seagrasses.
- **Marine Animals:** Animals are eukaryotic and multicellular organisms devoid of rigid cell walls. Their food is provided by other organisms since they are heterotrophs, unable to produce their own. Even sessile animals, except adult sponges, are able to move. Invertebrates are animals without backbones, and they make up the vast majority of species. Vertebrates have backbones.

**Lower Invertebrates**

- **Sponges:** The simplest of multicellular animals are the sponges. In addition, their cells exhibit little differentiation and specialization, and they lack tissues, organs, or a nervous system. Their growth forms and colours may vary, as they are asymmetrical and sessile.
- **Cnidarians:** There are four classes in the phylum Cnidaria- Hydrozoa, Scyphozoa, Cubozoa and Anthozoa. The body of a cnidarian is symmetrical, with its mouth forming the center of the body. In cnidaria, benthic polyps and pelagic medusas are the two basic body types.
- **Ctenophora:** Ctenophores are small, transparent, and radially symmetric. Tentacles of ctenophores are lined with adhesive cells and are used to catch prey. Many ctenophores are iridescent in the daytime and glow at night; they are believed to use their bioluminescence to attract mates or scare predators.

- **Platyhelminthes (Flatworms):** These worms have flattened bodies. The head and the posterior end of the animals show bilateral symmetry. Depending on their species, some flatworms are free-surviving while others are parasitic.
- **Nematodes (Round Worms):** Nematodes are the most abundant animals on the planet, and in some sediments, they can reach densities of up to 4,400,000 individuals/$m^2$. Both ends of their body are tapered, giving them a cylindrical appearance. Hermaphrodites constitute the majority.
- **Annelids (Segmented Worms):** Annelids possess an internal and external division of their bodies into repeated segments. This structure, coupled with a hydrostatic skeleton, allows enhanced mobility for these worms. Among marine annelids, polychaetes are the most common, living in a variety of habitats, such as rocks, mud, under rocks, in cracks, and in tubes they build for themselves. Several of them are mobile or errant, but others are sedentary.
- **Bryozoans:** Bryozoans belong to the Lophophorate group. There is no distinguishable head-on Lophophorate, but they are bilaterally symmetric. Lophophores are composed of ciliated tentacles that surround the mouth, and are used for feeding and gas exchange. The bryozoans are sessile and can be found on various types of seaweeds as well as in shallow waters.

**Higher Invertebrates**

- **Molluscs:** Molluscs occupy a diverse range of habitats and have soft bodies covered in calcium carbonate shells. Their body is divided into two major parts: the head-foot region comprises the head, mouth, sensory organs, and the foot, which functions as a locomotion apparatus. The radula is a tissue ribbon containing teeth used for scraping, piercing, tearing and cutting. Molluscs other than bivalves lack such a toothy structure.
- **Arthropods:** Arthropods are one of the most varied groups of animals, including terrestrial insects and account for 75% of all animal species. Chitin is the main component of the exoskeleton of arthropods, which provides protection and a way for muscles to attach. An arthropod's nervous system is highly developed, and its sense organs are extremely sophisticated. There are two major groups of marine arthropods: the chelicerates and the mandibulates.
- **Echinoderms:** Skins with spines are called Echinodermata. Animals belonging to this phylum include urchins, sea stars and sea cucumbers. Their ecological habitats range from shallow to deep sea. They have great regeneration abilities.

- **Tunicates:** Tunicates have a cellulose-like covering that covers their entire body, making them essentially sessile animals. They belong to the phylum Chordata. Usually round or cylindrical, sea squirts are sessile tunicates. Salps and larvaceans inhabit open ocean waters as pelagic tunicates.

**Marine Fishes:** Fish are vertebrates that have a series of bones and cartilage that support their spine and protect their muscles. Commercially harvested fish are used as food for human consumption and livestock feed, as well as fertilizers and other products.

Phylogenetic analysis of fishes identifies five main groups:

Hagfishes and lampreys are two of the most primitive animals, both lacking jaws and paired fins. Sharks, rays and relatives are cartilaginous fishes with cartilage-based skeletons. Ray-finned fishes possess bony skeletons, making them one of the most diverse groups of fishes. The lobe-finned fishes (Actinistia and Dipnoi) have a bony skeleton, with some of their fins having skeletal extensions. Their ancestors are land vertebrates [1].

**Marine Reptiles:** Reptiles are ectotherms and poikilotherms. Coldblooded creatures have a varying metabolic rate and level of activity, becoming sluggish in cold weather. Both land and water reptiles have adapted to survive on land and in water. As they eliminate waste efficiently while conserving water, their kidneys allow them to survive in dry and salty environments. Their skin generally lacks glands and is covered with scales, which minimizes water loss. Crocodiles, Sea turtles, Marine Iguanas and Sea Snakes are a few examples of reptiles.

**Marine Birds:** Despite changing temperatures in the environment, birds, also known as homeotherms, maintain a constant body temperature. The marine environment is home to about 250 species of birds among the 8,000 that exist. The flying skills, feeding mechanisms, and ability to live away from the land of seabirds differ greatly because they are descendants of different terrestrial bird groups. Large colonies of seabirds protect from predators, which is the reason why they are commonly found nesting together.

**Marine Mammals:** Mammals are members of the phylum Chordata and the class Mammalia. Oceans provide the majority of all of the food for marine mammals. For maintaining body temperature in water, marine mammals have a layer of insulating hair or blubber under their skin, as heat is lost more quickly than in air. Marine adaptations have evolved for three distinct orders of mammals. Sea otters, polar bears and seals fall into the Carnivora order, and sea cows (manatees and dugongs) fall into the Sirenia order. Whales, dolphins and porpoises are included in the Cetacean group.

## THREATS TO MARINE BIODIVERSITY

• **Habitat destruction:** Biodiversity loss is mainly caused by habitat destruction worldwide [5, 12, 13]. Lack of suitable habitat can lead to local extinction when there is no other suitable habitat nearby. By dividing large, continuous habitats into smaller patches of a smaller total area, habitat fragmentation can lead to smaller populations, which are more susceptible to genetic decline and local extinction. Habitat loss and fragmentation are often caused by human activities, especially in shallow coastal areas. Some examples of human intervention are:

(a) Fishing and aquaculture activities

(b) Coastal Development

(c) Tourism and recreation

(d) Climate change due to anthropogenic activities

- **Introduced species:** An introduced species is a species that has been moved by humans outside of its historic range, also called an exotic or alien species. The world has been home to thousands of marine species. It is possible to introduce microorganisms either intentionally or by accident via many types of vectors, including attachment to ships' hulls, inside ballast water of ships, release from aquariums, transit through man-made canals (e.g. the Suez Canal), and movement with various aquaculture products, among others.
- Native communities can be affected by invasive species in several ways, such as by competing for resources, preying on native species, spreading diseases, causing extinctions, and reducing biodiversity. Human activities may also be affected by invasive species.
- **Marine pollution:** A pollutant is something that is introduced into or exists in the environment, which can lead to harm. Pollutants emitted repeatedly or continuously or substances with very long persistence, constitute chronic pollution. Agricultural pesticides, for example, are a form of chronic pollution because they are found in the environment. An oil spill caused by the grounding of an oil tanker, for example, is an example of acute pollution, which occurs suddenly and usually severely. The term "point source pollution" describes pollution that originates from a single source, such as sewage discharge pipes. The impact of many septic systems in a watershed, for example, is a non-point source of pollution. Toxic substances (toxin substances), oil, plastic, and nutrients (eutrophication) are some of the factors contributing to marine pollution.

## BIOTECHNOLOGY IN THE OCEAN

Our ability to rationally search for active natural compounds and other novel biotechnologies is enabled by the study of biological systems in which there is a direct link between marine organisms' challenges and biotechnologies. The researchers have been able to develop effective methods for preventing marine biofouling and identifying new lead compounds through this approach [14]. Biological approaches are applied to marine organisms to harness them for a variety of commercial purposes. Biotechnology in the marine environment involves a combination of three traditional marine disciplines - ocean science, marine biology, and marine engineering - and the modern fields of molecular biology, genomics, and proteomics. Aside from offering trade routes, the oceans also provide food, aid in energy production (oil and gas), and provide recreation. Overfishing, habitat loss, boat traffic, pollution and climate change threaten the health of our ocean ecosystems. Many human activities can cause this problem, including converting coastal habitats for other purposes, nonpoint pollution, airborne pollutants, disease-causing bacteria, marine debris, ballast water, and invasive species. As part of the ongoing monitoring of ocean and coastal ecosystems, marine biotechnology has helped establish standard practices and procedures and guide management decisions about the ocean and coastal use. The desired information is collected using multiple means, including planes, ships, moored instruments, drifters, gliders, submersibles, remotely operated vehicles (ROV), and satellites. IOOS (Integrated Ocean Observing System) and GOOAS (Global Ocean Observing System) are two systems that keep track of oceanographic data. Counting populations of marine organisms is done with optical and sonic probes. In the past few years, advances in molecular biology, ecology, and environmental engineering have opened up opportunities to modify organisms so that their basic biological processes are more efficient and can degrade chemical compounds and greater volumes of waste materials [15, 16]. Some of the more pressing issues revolve around the extraction of renewable energy resources, and the elimination of industrial waste. This should prove to be particularly true in relation to marine systems, which will likely face stricter regulations as they become subject to increasing anthropogenic degradation. Such regulations will almost certainly require new regulatory frameworks, and novel biotechnological approaches. Existing biotechnological methods are already proving just how effective these approaches can be at dealing with both of these concerns in most terrestrial environments. Given their existing potential for marine applications, there is good reason to believe that they will play a similar role in the future of marine ecological communities [15-17].

## CONCLUSION

The future of marine biology and biotechnology depends much on the possibilities of a cleaner and sustainable environment that promotes the well-being of the animals, plants and humans living in this environment. Biotechnology will become a way to sustainably keep the ecosystem functioning. Biotechnological experiments are currently being conducted to develop methods of gene mapping, environmental DNA testing and genetic based regulations as well as ways of monitoring detrimental effects of marine invasive species. The ocean is a vast resource that has tremendous amounts of microbial life. Through advances in science, it will be possible for us to understand this microbial ecology and improve our lives through new bio-technology. Slowly but steadily, marine biotechnology is entering a new dawn. In the coming years, we'll see increased public engagement with marine biotechnology through support of universities and NGOs, as well as investment from private industry into business ventures. Despite the difficulties that marine biotechnology will face, the benefits of successful implementation are so compelling that we must see these challenges as an opportunity to tackle innovation in order to reap success. Through the use of many emerging technologies in robotics, computer modelling and simulation, synthetic biology, nanotechnology, and other related fields, the sea is a bounty waiting to be harvested. The question is whether or not marine biotechnology will sink or swim—the next few years will tell.

## REFERENCES

1. Gephart JA, Golden CD, Asche F, Belton B, Brugere C, Froehlich HE, Fry JP, Halpern BS, Hicks CC, Jones RC, Klinger DH, Little DC, McCauley DJ, Thilsted SH, Troell M, Allison EH. Scenarios for Global Aquaculture and its Role in Human Nutrition. Rev Fish Sci Aquacult 2021; 29: 122-138.
2. Herlihy T, Sifneos JC, Hughes RM, Peck DV, Mitchell RM. Relation of Lotic Fish and Benthic Macroinvertebrate condition Indices to Environmental Factors across the Conterminous USA. Ecol Indicat 2020; 112: 105958.
3. Gui JF, Zhou L, Li XY. Rethinking Fish Biology and Biotechnologies in the challenge Era for Burgeoning Genome Resources and Strengthening Food Security. Water Biol Secur 2022; article in press.
4. Tickner D, Opperman JJ, Abell R. *et al.* Bending the Curve of Global Freshwater Biodiversity Loss: An Emergency Recovery Plan. BioScience 2020; 70: 330-342.
5. Schinegger R, Palt M, Segurado P, Schmutz S. Untangling the Effects of Multiple Human Stressors and their Impacts on Fish Assemblages in European Running Waters. Sci Total Environ 2016; 573: 1079-1088.
6. Rocky DN, Steinberg PD. Linking Marine Biology and Biotechnology. Current Opinion in Biotechnology 2002; 13 (3): 244-248.
7. Cogan CB, Todd BJ, Lawton P, Noji TT. The Role of Marine Habitat Mapping in Ecosystem-based Management. ICES Journal of Marine Science 2009; 66: 2033-2042.
8. Copeland A, Edinger E, Devillers R, Bell T, *et al.* Marine Habitat Mapping in Support of Marine Protected Area management in a Subarctic fjord: Gilbert Bay, Labrador, Canada. Journal of Coastal Conservation 2013; 17(2): 225-237.
9. Foster-Smith RL, Sotheran IS. Mapping Marine Benthic Biotopes using Acoustic Ground Discrimination systems. International Journal of Remote Sensing 2003; 24(13): 2761-2784.

10. Foody G. Assessing the Accuracy of Remotely Sensed Data: Principles and Practices. The Photogrammetric Record 2010; 25(130): 204-205.
11. Goodman J, Ustin SL. Classification of benthic Composition in a Coral Reef Environment using Spectral Unmixing. Journal of Applied Remote Sensing 2007; 1(1): 11501.
12. Day J, Fernandes L, Lewis A, De'Ath G *et al.* The Representative Areas Program for Protecting Biodiversity in the Great Barrier Reef World Heritage Area. Proceedings of the Ninth International Coral Reef Symposium 2002; 2: 687-696.
13. Attwood C. Putting into Practice the Ecosystem approach to Fisheries. Business & Economics, 76pp. Food and Agriculture Organization of the United Nations.
14. Chen B, Wan C, Mehmood MA, Chang JS, Bai F, Zhao X. Manipulating Environmental Stresses and Stress Tolerance of Microalgae for Enhanced Production of Lipids and Value-added Products–a Review. Bioresour Technol 2017; 244: 1198-1206.
15. Datta A, Mukherjee D, Jessup L. Understanding Commercialization of Technological Innovation: Taking Stock and moving forward. R D Manag 2014; 45: 215-249.
16. Barbier M, Reitz A, Pabortsava K, Wölfl AC, Hahn T, Whoriskey F. Ethical Recommendations for Ocean Observation. Adv Geosci 2018; 45: 343-361.
17. Carroll AR, Copp BR, Davis RA, Keyzers RA, Prinsep MR. Marine Natural Products. Nat Prod Rep 2019; 36: 122-173.

**Corresponding author: Dr Amit Gupta, Associate Professor, Department of Biotechnology, Graphic Era (Deemed to be) University, Dehradun, India.**
**Email id: dr.amitgupta.bt@geu.ac.in**

Pages: 75-82
**Emerging Environmental Contaminants and Global Healthcare Systems**
*Editors:* **Prof. (Dr.) Shyam Narain Pandey; Murtaza Abid**
**Prof. (Dr.) Syed Rais Haider; Dr. Sabiha Kazmi; Dr. Mohd. Zahid Rizvi**
*ISBN:* **978-81-959169-2-4**
*Edition:* **2023**
*Published by:* **Discovery Publishing House, New Delhi (India)**

# Microbes in the Environment

**Kaniska and Amit Gupta**

## ABSTRACT

*In literature, microbes are generally called as Ubiquitous, it means they are reported and found everywhere in the environment. In other words, these microorganisms may directly have benefitted or harmful to the environment or showing metabolic activities of microbes with plants and animals (usage in production of food material and biotechnological processes). Till date, most of the microbial species are not identified yet, as scientists were not able to estimate the biodiversity of microbes due to problem in conventional taxonomic method (species that are similar to the hierarchy order). Most of the microbes present in the environment cause disease to humans and plants. Some of the microbes (bacteria, fungi and protozoa) helps in cleaning the environment recycle of the primary element (nitrogen, oxygen and carbon), decomposition of the organic matter, bioremediation of the sewage water, degradation of plastics and waste etc. In this chapter, we discuss about the role of microbes in the environment.*

***Keywords:*** *Ubiquitous, conventional taxonomic method, Bioremediation, Decomposition and Degradation.*

## INTRODUCTION

Microbes are small organisms that cannot be seen with the naked eyes but these microorganisms are reported in a wide range. In general, these microbes consist of protozoans, viruses, bacteria, fungi, and algae (blue green algae or cyanobacteria). So, these microbes may directly or indirectly

**Department of Biotechnology, Graphic Era (Deemed to be) University, Dehradun, (India)**

contribute to the quality of human life. In literature, microbes are found in any kind of habitat such as aquatic, terrestrial, high and cold temperature area, atmosphere, high salt environment etc. So, there is large diversity of microbes are reported in the environment [1, 2]. One of the most familiar example is seen in terrestrial environmental microbes are reported in soil which consists of 11000 species approximately of bacteria, fungi, actinomycetes, protozoa and some viruses. So, these soil derived bacteria usually degrade organic matter, helps in fixing the content of nitrogen and also helpful in the process of nitrification (*Nitrobacter* and *Nitrosomonas*). In addition, actinomycete (prokaryotic in nature) forms asexual spores and mycelium like fungi, maintain equilibrium in soil, helps in production of antibiotic (*streptomycin* and *tetracycline*), degrade cellulose humus, hemicellulos and lignin. In contrast, fungi species are reported in soil and bears fruiting body, and mostly club shaped structure, degrade proteins, nucleic acid (ammonification) and kills nematodes. Similarly, algae (unicellular and filamentous) provide oxygen to plants and produce polysaccharides [3, 4]. Aquatic habitat microflora is mainly divided into three communities i.e. planktons, heptobenthos, and herpobenthos. Microbes can survive in extreme high temperature called thermophile e.g. *Bacillus stereothermophilus, Bacillus subtilis and* red algae Cyanidium. The microbes that can survive in cold temperature (-20°C or below) are known to be Psychrophile e.g. *Pseudomonas, Sphingomonas* and *Arthrobacter species.* Microbes are medically important for the manufacturing of drugs, vaccines and antibiotics which helps the human beings for their treatment against infectious diseases [5, 6]. So, these microbes played a symbiotic role with the environment derived bacteria which is present in the human or animal intestine and helpful in nutrient digestion and may helpful to produce essential vitamins. In addition, some of the microbes are also present on the surface of the skin which may protect from several infections. In short, these microbes are so important to the environment, but everything have advantages and their disadvantages [1-6].

Day by day population is increasing and there is need of more crops yield due to which more decomposition of organic matter happens and release more nitrogen and carbon source to the environment. Though microbes cleaning the environment but release of more $CO_2$ in environment can be a major cause of global warming [7, 8]. Microbes can harm humans in great extent in the form of diseases which are mainly caused through bacteria, viruses and fungi. Not only humans but plants also get affected by some fungi and viruses. So, there are many reasons to study microbes and their morphology for the drastic change in climate, new species was generating that affecting human health. Some of the most significant role of microbes in the environment are:

**Decomposition:** Decomposition is the process of breaking down of complex substances to its simpler form. The major element present in plant and animals is carbon which is an organic matter. Some of the microbes like bacteria and fungi decompose the organic matter present in dead plants and animals. These organic matter mixes with the soil and convert into simple substances, provide essential nutrients to the soil. The process of humification and mineralization occurs during decomposition. In humification the substance act as a reservoir of the nutrients (colloidal in nature) to form humus. Further the process of mineralisation degrades the humus to inorganic nutrients required for the growth of the plant [9, 10]. The most important factors required for the process of decomposition is the availability of oxygen, moisture of the soil, temperature and climatic conditions. If there were no microbes in the soil, then the dead plants and animal's wastes will keep increasing making the environment unclean or dirty e.g. *Thiothrix, Thiobacillus, Chlorobium species.*

**Improves soil fertility:** Some of the microbes present in the soil helps to fix nitrogen gas from the atmosphere to form nitrogen derived compounds. Using the same land for cultivation again and again which is responsible for depleting the concentration of the nutrients. All plants need nutrients for their development. The most familiar example is seen in leguminous crop plants which have special types of roots that have nodules in which rhizobium nitrogen fixing bacteria is present and provide nitrogen to the plant. *Mycorrhizae,* symbiotic relationship between fungi and plant may increase the uptake and mobility of phosphorous to the soil, protects roots of the soil from toxic metals and pathogens that are harmful [11, 12].

**Sewage water Treatment:** Sewage is the domestic and household waste (hospital waste, washing clothes, human excreta etc.). Microbes are used to remove organic waste and pollutants. In water there are many substances present like heavy metals, oils artificial fertilizers, organic matter, and detergents which have to be removed for cleaning of water. Firstly, all the larger objects like stones, sand and rocks are removed physically by the Grit chamber. In primary treatment, the waste is filtered and sedimented (heavy substance settles down when treated with Alum, aluminium oxides and chlorine). Further, secondary treatment also known as biological treatment where the substance transfers to the aeration tank or chamber which supply continuous oxygen. Flocs (bacterial associated with fungal filaments) are formed when bacteria are added to the aeration tank. The bacteria present in the water digest all the organic matter with the continuous supply of oxygen and decreases the BOD (biological oxygen demand). After, the flocs transfer to the secondary settling tank in which flocs settled (activated sludge). The process is repeated until the water get clean and some of the anaerobic bacteria digest the remaining flocs and release some energy and methane, $H_2S$ and $CO_2$ (biogas) [13, 14]. The polluted water gets cleaned and can now be released to the rivers e.g. methanogens.

**Extraction of metals from ores:** Minerals can also be extracted from the ores with the help of microbes, the term known to be bioleaching (microbial ore leaching). In the Leaching process, bacteria play an important role to revive the ore oxidizer (ferric iron). The bacterial species mainly oxidizes the ferrous iron and sulphur. Further, bacteria produce energy and reduces oxygen from the water. Basically using of microbes for metal extraction is safer and make the environment clean from toxicity [15]. Species helps bioleaching example bacteria (*Acidithiobacillus ferroxidants*), fungi (*Aspergillus Niger).*

**Bioremediation to clean oil spills:** Bioremediation is the process which breakdown the oil spill components with the help of microbes. These microbes absorb the toxic components present in the oil spill that can harm aquatic life. The process of layering of oil due to oil spill is called eutrophication which causes absence of oxygen [16] e.g. *Pseudomonas putida.*

**Degradation of plastic waste:** Now days, plastics were used in every house but these plastics and polythenes can cause serious issue to the environment [17]. Microbes obtain nutrients from the plastic by the enzymatic degradation process. Plastic material can be degraded by the two methods either by aerobic or anaerobic conditions. In aerobic condition, bacteria use oxygen as an electron acceptor and convert the complex organic chemicals present in plastics to the simpler form (end product $CO_2$ and water) e.g. *Bacillus cereus, Streptomyces Species, Phanerochae chrysosporium* etc.

## HARMFUL IMPACT OF MICROBES TO THE ENVIRONMENT

Microbes that affect and caused severe infection are known as pathogen. The only microbe that not caused the disease are algae and archaebacteria. This disease can even cause death of the organisms. Some of the bacterial disease which is mainly transmitted from water, air, and contact. Various bacterial diseases (Table 10.1).

Some of the fungi cause skin infection like ringworm, yeast infection and athlete foot. Some of the microbes also cause infection to the plant's necrosis, tumours, soft rot etc.

Similarly, viral disease is mainly transmitted through contact or air. The most familiar examples of viral diseases as shown in Table 10.2.

**Table 10.1: Bacterial Diseases**

| S.No. | Disease | Mode of Transmission | Causative Agent | Symptoms |
|---|---|---|---|---|
| 1. | Cholera | Water borne | *Vibrio cholera* | Diarrhoea |
| 2. | Anthrax | Air borne | *Bacillus anthrax* | Affect respiratory system |
| 3. | Tetanus | Rusted iron | *Clostridium tetani* | Problem of lock jaw |
| 4. | Syphilis | STI (sexually transmitted infection) | *Treponema pallidum* | Organ damage |
| 5. | Pneumonia | Air borne | *Streptococcus pneumonia* | Infect lungs (fluid filled alveoli) |
| 6. | Typhoid | Water borne | *Salmonella typhi* | Intestinal perforation |
| 7. | Tuberculosis | Air borne | *Mycobacterium tuberculosis* | Cough , joint pain |
| 8. | Gonorrhoea | STI | *Neisseria gonorrhoea* | Infection in reproductive system |
| 9. | Diphtheria | Air borne | *Corynebacterium diphtheriae* | Cough, Horse voice |
| 10. | Pertussis | Air borne | *Bordetella pertussis* | Constant coughing |
| 11. | Leprosy | Contact | *Mycobacterium leprae* | White patches on the body with puss |
| 12. | Botulism | Water borne | *Clostridium botulinum* | Affect the nervous system |

**Table 10.2: Viral Diseases**

| S.No. | Disease | Mode of Transmission | Causative Agent | Symptoms |
|---|---|---|---|---|
| 1. | Hepatitis | Blood transfusion, oral faecal route, STI | Hepatitis virus (A, B, C, D) | Liver cirrhosis, loss of appetite |
| 2. | AIDS | STI | HIV (human immune deficiency virus) | Low immunity |
| 3. | Rabies | Dog bite | *Rhabdovirus* | Hallucination, excessive, salvation paralysis |
| 4. | Poliomyelitis | Water borne | *Polio virus* | Attacks nervous system |
| 5. | Influenza | Air borne | *Myxovirus* | Sneezing, headache, pneumonia |
| 6. | Chicken pox | Contact (touch) | *Vorcella zoster* | Abdomen pain, red colour scabs on the body |
| 7. | Mumps | Infection of parotoid gland Air borne | *Paramyxovirus* | Inflammation of parotoid gland |
| 8. | Measles | Air borne | *Rubeola virus* | Face, neck scabs |
| 9. | Small pox | Air borne, contact | *Variola virus* | Irradicated all over the body |
| 10. | Chikungunya | Vector | *Chikungunya virus* | Extreme joint pain |
| 11. | Dengue | Vector | *Arbovirus* | Internal bleeding, low platelet count |
| 12. | Corona | Air borne, contact | *SARS-COV-2* | Fever, cough, loss of taste or smell and tiredness |

## CONCLUSION

There will be no doubt about how microbes related to the environment, but there must be a clarity of how microbe react and how they impact our life. Scientists were still studying and searching for the upcoming variation in the microbes due to evolution.

## REFERENCES


1. Adeleke R, Dames JF. *Kalaharituber pfeilii* and associated Bacterial Interactions. South Afr J Bot 2014; 90: 68-73.
2. Bang C, Dagan T, Deines P, Dubilier N, Duschl WJ, Fraune S, *et al*. Metaorganisms in Extreme Environments: Do Microbes Play a Role in Organismal adaptation. Zoology 2018; 127: 1-19.
3. Berg G, Smalla K. Plant Species and Soil Type Cooperatively Shape the Structure and Function of Microbial Communities in the Rhizosphere. FEMS Microbiol Ecol 2009; 68: 1-13.
4. Cheeseman JM. The evolution of Halophytes, Glycophytes and Crops, and its Implications for Food Security under Saline Conditions. New Phytol 2015; 206: 557-570.
5. El-Deeb B, Fayez K, Gherbawy Y. Isolation and Characterization of Endophytic Bacteria from *Plectranthus tenuiflorus* Medicinal Plant in Saudi Arabia Desert and their Antimicrobial Activities. J Plant Interact 2013; 8, 56-64.
6. Hanna AL, Youssef HH, Amer WM, Monib M, Fayez M, Hegazi NA. Diversity of Bacteria Nesting the Plant Cover of North Sinai Deserts. Egypt J Adv Res 2013; 4: 13-26.
7. Briones MJI, Poskitt J, Ostle N. Influence of Warming and Enchytraeid Activities on Soil $CO_2$ and $CH_4$ Fluxes. Soil Biol Biochem 2004; 36: 1851-1859.
8. Jenkinson DS, Adams DE, Wild A. Model estimates of $CO_2$ Emissions from Soil in Response to Global Warming. Nature 1991; 351: 304-306.
9. Anisimov OA, Nelson FE, Pavlov AV. Predictive Scenarios of Permafrost Development under Conditions of Global Climate Change in the XXI Century. Earth Cryology 1999; 3: 15-25.
10. Schlesinger WH, Lichter J. Limited Carbon Storage in Soil and Litter of Experimental Forest Plots under Increased $CO_2$. Nature 2001; 411: 466-469.
11. Antoniadis V, Koutroubas SD, Fotiadis S (2015) Nitrogen, Phosphorus, and Potassium Availability in Manure- and Sewage Sludge–Applied Soil. Commun Soil Sci Plant Anal 46: 393-404.
12. Bergkvist P, Jarvis N, Berggren D, Carlgren K. Long-term Effects of Sewage Sludge Applications on Soil Properties, Cadmium Availability and Distribution in Arable Soil. Agric Ecosyst Environ 2003; 97: 167-179.
13. Bloem E, Albihn A, Elving J, Hermann L, Lehmann L, Sarvi M, Schaaf T, Schick J, Turtola E, Ylivainio K. Contamination of Organic Nutrient Sources with Potentially Toxic Elements, Antibiotics and Pathogen Microorganisms in relation to P Fertilizer Potential and Treatment Options for the Production of Sustainable Fertilizers: A Review. Sci Total Environ 2017; 607: 225-242.
14. Andriamananjara A, Rabeharisoa L, Prud'homme L, Morel C. Drivers of Plant-availability of Phosphorus from Thermally Conditioned Sewage Sludge as assessed by Isotopic Labelling. Front Nutr 2016; 3:19.

15. Börjesson G, Kirchmann H, Kätterer T. Four Swedish long-term Field Experiments with Sewage Sludge Reveal a Limited Effect on Soil Microbes and on Metal uptake by Crops. J Soils Sediments 2014; 14: 164-177.
16. Abbasnezhad H, Gray M, Foght JM. Influence of Adhesion on Aerobic Biodegradation and Bioremediation of Liquid Hydrocarbons. Appl Microbiol Biotechnol 2011; 92: 653-675.
17. Das MP, Kumar S. An Approach to Low-density Polyethylene Biodegradation by *Bacillus amyloliquefaciens*. 3 Biotech 2015; 5: 81-86.

**Corresponding author: Dr Amit Gupta, Associate Professor, Department of Biotechnology, Graphic Era (Deemed to be) University, Dehradun, India.**
**Email id: dr.amitgupta.bt@geu.ac.in**

Pages: 83-87
**Emerging Environmental Contaminants and Global Healthcare Systems**
*Editors:* **Prof. (Dr.) Shyam Narain Pandey; Murtaza Abid**
**Prof. (Dr.) Syed Rais Haider; Dr. Sabiha Kazmi; Dr. Mohd. Zahid Rizvi**
*ISBN:* **978-81-959169-2-4**
*Edition:* **2023**
*Published by:* **Discovery Publishing House, New Delhi (India)**

# Ocean Acidification and its Impacts

**Navleen Kaur, *Harmanpreet Kaur**
****Vidhi N. Pansuriya, Amit Gupta**

## ABSTRACT

*Ocean acidification is a deadly issue over a decade. The alteration in pH of ocean water due to anthropogenic activities has led to distortion of marine ecosystem. The alteration in chemistry of ocean water which may result into a change in the carbonate system of aquatic lifestyle. Excess dissolution of carbon dioxide in water bodies and lowering of pH is responsible for causing ocean acidification. Due to this acidification, it may be directly impact on our ecosystem as scientists have witnessed some irreversible changes which are reported in the marine life, and this can also lead to loss of habitat. According to data, the surface ocean's acidity has increased by more than 34% since 1852, and it might quadruple by 2300 as a result of rising* $CO_2$ *emissions from a growing human population. Despite the fact that research on the protracted ecological implications of acidification in the oceans is still in its early stages, radical changes in species distributions and species richness in marine food webs may occur at several trophic levels. This article will discuss about the phenomenon of acidification of ocean and its effects on marine ecosystem.*

***Keywords:*** *Anthropogenic activities, marine ecosystem, habitat loss, acidification and ecological impacts.*

## INTRODUCTION

Our atmosphere is comprised of 0.4% of carbon dioxide i.e., 412.5 parts per million. The feasible and healthy amount of $CO_2$ to be present in

**Department of Sciences, Govt. Mohindra College, Patiala, Punjab (India)**
***Department of Biotechnology, Graphic Era (Deemed to be) University, Dehradun (India)**
****Infinity Pathology Laboratory, Katargam, Surat (Gujarat)**

ocean is 387 ppm. No doubt, carbon dioxide is one of the essential gases comprising air of our atmosphere, but excess of everything is threatening. Ocean acidification is the phenomenon of increase in amount of carbon dioxide (beyond its sustainable limit) of ocean water resulting to decrease in pH level. During the industrial revolution, the pH of the ocean plummeted from 8.2 to 7.7. Since, the pH scale which is logarithmic just similar to Richter scale for evaluating and measuring earthquakes, a 0.1 fall in pH may not seem like much. If present carbon dioxide emissions continue, seawater levels might decrease another 122 percent by the end of the century. This would culminate in an ocean that is more corrosive than any that has existed in the previous 20 million years or longer. Hypercapnia is a condition in which the partial pressure of $CO_2$ ($pCO_2$) in seawater is elevated or increased, resulting in a decrease in the absorption rate of calcium carbonate ($CaCO_3$), which directly impacts calcification rates and disrupts the physiology of the acid-base (metabolic) pathway [1, 2]. Many calcifying species are endangered by manmade $CO_2$ uptake in the Mediterranean, as well as changes in diversification, trophic relationships, and other ecological processes, according to recent research. The most attention has been paid to tropical coral reefs and planktonic coccolithophores. Additional key species, mechanisms other than calcification, or the expected ecosystem-level repercussions of rising marine $pCO_2$ levels over the next 100 years are all unknown.

### *Ocean Acidification and Ocean Carbonate System*

Ocean acidification is defined as the phenomenon of lowering the pH of ocean water due to excessive dissolution of $CO_2$. The inorganic carbon system, which is primarily responsible for controlling the pH of seawater, is one of the most important chemical equilibria in the ocean. At a pH of 8.1, $HCO_3$ 2- makes up 89 percent of the carbon in the solution, CO3 makes up 10%, and dissolved $CO_2$ makes up only 0.6 percent. When $CO_2$ dissolves in seawater, $H_2CO_3$ is produced. The bulk of the $H_2CO_3$ quickly dissociates into hydrogen ion (H+) and $HCO_3$ 2-. Following that, a hydrogen ion can react with a $CO_3$ 2- molecule to produce bicarbonate. As a consequence, delivering $CO_2$ to seawater enhances $H_2CO_3$, $HCO_3$, and H+ concentrations while decreasing $CO_3$ concentration and raising pH. These reactions in seawater have well-understood thermodynamics and are completely reversible. The current $CO_2$ level in the atmosphere is 110 parts per million higher than the pre-industrial level (283 parts per million), whereas the average surface ocean pH has fallen by 0.2 units, suggesting a 31% increase in [H+] [3,4]. According to IPCC emission estimates, average surface ocean pH by the end of the century might be 0.2-0.5 pH units lower than pre-industrial values.

### Effects of Ocean Acidification

***Fishes:*** On the West Coast, both aquaculture facilities and natural ecosystems have seen near-total oyster failures in the recent past. Natural upwelling episodes that deliver low pH, aragonite-undersaturated waters to nearshore areas, as well as other water quality changes, appear to be associated to these larval oyster deaths. On the West Coast, lower pH levels are common during intertidal occurrences, but a new study suggests that anthropogenic $CO_2$ is causing seasonal undersaturation. Low pH may induce oyster reproduction failure; however, further study is needed to differentiate suspected acidification effects from other risk factors such as repeated freshwater intrusion, disease development, or a lack of dissolved oxygen. Although it is too early to determine if ocean acidification is to blame for oyster failures, oyster industry experts believe it may play a part in the current situation, which is costing the business $100 million each year. Pteropods, sometimes known as "sea butterflies," are little aquatic organisms approximately the size of a pea.[5]. Pteropods are consumed by species as little as krill to as large as whales, and they feed juvenile salmon in the North Pacific. Pteropods are consumed by species as little as krill to as large as whales, and they feed juvenile salmon in the North Pacific.

***Marine flora:*** Plants and algae can benefit from acidic conditions. More carbon dioxide in the water is advantageous rather than detrimental to these organisms because they get their energy from a mixture of sunshine and carbon dioxide. Seagrasses grow in shallow waters that act as nursery for a variety of bigger fish and can support hundreds of species. They are, however, diminishing owing to a variety of reasons, most notably pollution pouring into coastal waters, and it is unclear if acidification can account for all of these losses. They are, however, diminishing owing to a variety of reasons, most notably pollution pouring into coastal waters, and it is unclear if acidification can account for all of these losses. Certain algae species flourish in increasingly acidic conditions as carbon dioxide levels rise. Coralline algae, on the other hand, which produce calcium carbonate skeletons and help in coral reef cementation, don't fare so well. Because it is more soluble than aragonite or ordinary calcite, most coralline algae species use high-magnesium calcite calcium carbonate in their shells. According to one study, coralline algae filled 92 percent less surface area in acidifying conditions, making room for other types of non-calcifying algae that can choke and kill coral reefs. When coral larvae are preparing to leave the plankton stage and undergo metamorphosis on a coral reef, they prefer to settle on coralline algae. Shells are produced by coccolithophores, a kind of microalgae (single-celled algae that floating and bloom in surface waters). These organisms' shells degraded with time, much like the shells of other shelled species, leaving them vulnerable to injury [6-9]. Longer-term studies found that a typical coccolithophore could multiply for 720 iterations, or around a year, underneath the warmer, more acidic conditions that will be the norm in 100 years. The population evolved strong shells as a result of their adaptation. It's conceivable that they just took longer to acclimatise, or that adaption varies by species or population.

***On human life:*** Changes in marine ecosystems will have an impact on human society, which relies on the commodities and services provided by these ecosystems [10-12]. Social impacts might include significant income drops, job and livelihood losses, and other indirect economic expenses.

If the following environmental services are diminished, they are likely to have socio-economic consequences:

- Ocean acidification has the potential to jeopardise food security. Marine species that are economically and ecologically significant will be harmed, albeit their responses may vary. Oysters and mussels are among the most threatened molluscs. On a business-as-usual (RCP8.6) $CO_2$ emissions trajectory, the worldwide yearly costs of mollusc loss from ocean acidification might reach US$120 billion by 2200.
- Corals, for example, insulate shorelines from storm surges and storms, protecting many island nations' sole liveable region. The annual worth of reefs' protective role in preventing loss of life, property damage, and erosion is estimated to be $8.9 billion.
- Ocean acidification's influence on marine habitats might have a significant impact on this business (e.g., coral reefs). The Great Barrier Reef Marine Park in Australia draws over 1.8 million visitors each year and earns the Australian economy approximately A$5.7 billion.
- As ocean acidification worsens, the ocean's ability to absorb $CO_2$ reduces. Oceans that are more acidic are less efficient in reducing climate change [15].

## CONCLUSION

The acidification of the water, like other climate changes, is a complex and intimidating task. Although the biological effects of ocean acidification on marine creatures are just now being recognised, the changes in seawater chemistry produced by $CO_2$ absorption in the atmosphere have been widely documented throughout the vast majority of the ocean. New technologies and breakthroughs, as well as coordinated, interdisciplinary initiatives combining biologists and researchers, experimentalists, and domain specialists, will be necessary to assess the consequences of ocean acidification on marine fauna and changes in ecosystem functioning. Nonetheless, there is enough evidence to conclude unambiguously that negative effects on certain marine species are inescapable, and that significant changes in marine ecosystems are projected during the next century.

## REFERENCES

1. Hoegh-Guldberg, O., Mumby, P.J., Hooten, A.J., Steneck, R.S., Greenfield, P., Gomez, E., Harvell, C.D., Sale, P.F., Edwards, A.J., Caldeira, K., Knowlton, N., Eakin, C.M., Iglesias-Prieto, R., Muthiga, N., Bradbury, R.H., Dubi, A. and Hatziolos, M.E. (2007). Coral Reefs Under Rapid Climate Change and Ocean Acidification. Science, 318(5857), 1737-1742. doi:10.1126/science.1152509.

2. Boyd Philip, W. (2011). Beyond Ocean Acidification., 4(5), 273-274. doi:10.1038/ngeo1150.
3. Ekstrom Julia A., Suatoni Lisa, Cooley Sarah, R. Pendleton Linwood, H., Waldbusser George, G., Cinner Josh, E., Ritter Jessica, Langdon Chris, van Hooidonk Ruben, Gledhill Dwight, Wellman Katharine, Beck Michael, W., Brander Luke, M., Rittschof Dan, Doherty Carolyn, Edwards Peter, E.T. and Portela Rosimeiry (2015). Vulnerability and Adaptation of US Shellfisheries to Ocean Acidification. Nature Climate Change, 5(3), 207-214. doi:10.1038/nclimate2508.
4. Kristy, J. Kroeker Rebecca, L. Kordas, Ryan N. Crim and Gerald G. Singh (2010). Meta-analysis Reveals Negative yet Variable Effects of Ocean Acidification on Marine Organisms. , 13(11), 1419-1434. doi:10.1111/j.1461-0248.2010.01518. x.
5. Fabry, V.J., Seibel, B.A. Feely R.A. and Orr, J.C. (2008). Impacts of Ocean Acidification on Marine Fauna and Ecosystem Processes. ICES Journal of Marine Science, 65(3), 414-432. doi:10.1093/icesjms/fsn048.
6. Kroeker Kristy, J., Kordas Rebecca, L., Crim Ryan, Hendriks Iris, E., Ramajo Laura Singh, Gerald S., Duarte Carlos M. and Gattuso Jean-Pierre (2013). *Impacts of Ocean Acidification on Marine Organisms: Quantifying Sensitivities and Interaction with Warming. Global Change Biology, 19(6), 1884-1896.* doi:10.1111/gcb.12179.
7. Doney Scott, C., Fabry Victoria, J., Feely Richard, A. and Kleypas Joan, A. (2009). Ocean Acidification: The Other CO <sub/>2</sub> Problem. Annual Review of Marine Science, 1(1), 169-192. doi: 10.1146/annurev.marine.010908.163834.
8. John M. Guinotte and Victoria J. Fabry (2008). Ocean Acidification and its Potential Effects on Marine Ecosystems., 1134(none), 320-342. doi:10.1196/annals.1439.013.
9. Thomsen, J. *et al.* Bio geosciences 7, 3879-3891 (2010).
10. Dupont Sam and Pörtner Hans (2013). *Marine Science: Get ready for Ocean Acidification. Nature, 498(7455), 429-429.* doi:10.1038/498429a
11. Dupont Sam and Pörtner Hans (2013). Marine Science: Get ready for Ocean Acidification. Nature, 498(7455), 429-429. doi:10.1038/498429a.
12. Branch Trevor, A., D.E. Joseph Bonnie, M., Ray Liza J.; Wagner, Cherie A. (2013). *Impacts of Ocean Acidification on Marine Seafood. Trends in Ecology & Evolution, 28(3), 178-186.* doi: 10.1016/j.tree.2012.10.001.
13. Doney, Scott C.; Busch, D. Shallin; Cooley, Sarah R.; Kroeker, Kristy J. (2020). *The Impacts of Ocean Acidification on Marine Ecosystems and Reliant Human Communities. Annual Review of Environment and Resources, 45(1), annurev-environ-012320-083019.* doi:10.1146/annurev-environ-012320-083019
14. Parker, Laura; Ross, Pauline; O'Connor, Wayne; Pörtner, Hans; Scanes, Elliot; Wright, John (2013). *Predicting the Response of Molluscs to the Impact of Ocean Acidification. Biology, 2(2), 651-692.* doi:10.3390/biology2020651
15. Gazeau, Frederic; Parker, Laura M.; Comeau, Steeve; Gattuso, Jean-Pierre; Oâ Connor, Wayne A.; Martin, Sophie; Partner, Hans-Otto; Ross, Pauline M. (2013). *Impacts of Ocean Acidification on Marine shelled Molluscs. Marine Biology, 160(8), 2207-2245.* doi:10.1007/s00227-013-2219-3

---

**Corresponding author: Dr Amit Gupta, Associate Professor, Department of Biotechnology, Graphic Era (Deemed to be) University, Dehradun, India.**
**Email id: dr.amitgupta.bt@geu.ac.in**

Pages: 88-93
**Emerging Environmental Contaminants and Global Healthcare Systems**
*Editors:* **Prof. (Dr.) Shyam Narain Pandey; Murtaza Abid**
**Prof. (Dr.) Syed Rais Haider; Dr. Sabiha Kazmi; Dr. Mohd. Zahid Rizvi**
*ISBN:* **978-81-959169-2-4**
*Edition:* **2023**
*Published by:* **Discovery Publishing House, New Delhi (India)**

# Conception of Sustainable Development

**Lata Mehta, Mansi Kumari, Amit Gupta**

**ABSTRACT**

*The United Nations' Sustainable Development Goals include sustainable agriculture as a key component. Agriculture is the largest producer on the planet. It has been characterized as a typical top-down method since the green revolution. Pasture and agriculture cover over half of the planet's habitable land and supply residuals and food for a diverse range of organisms. Unsustainable methods, on the other hand, have a significant negative impact on the environment and people. The topic of sustainability has added complexity and alternatives to what was previously a very easy process of innovation, operational agriculture, leading to mistrust models. However, the next stage of development has numerous challenges in terms of economic development.*

***Keywords:*** *Sustainable agriculture, farmers and nutrients.*

## INTRODUCTION

In literature, sustainable agriculture means the ability of a farm to produce or generate food for animals including humans, without showing any damage to our ecosystem. The basic goal of sustainable agriculture is to meet the demands of society or countries in terms of food, including textiles, without jeopardizing future generations' ability to meet their own needs. Sustainable agriculture aims to achieve three key goals in its work: environmental health, economic profitability, and social and economic equity [1]. The term "sustainability" is directly applied to agriculture and considers a holistic and long-term approach in terms of business on-farm which means

**Department of Life Sciences, Graphic Era Deemed to be University, Dehradun (India)**

maximizing stability about economic and environmental level, equity, and health of the farm and its business. In other words, sustainability mainly focuses and is applied to business practices and their process, rather than a specific type of food fibered. One of the examples is seen in the case of agriculture where there is a huge demand to increase the rate of sustainability in agriculture at the global level. Due to intensive knowledge and application of sustainability, this may create some challenges and opportunities in agriculture [1, 2]. Farmers often need to take a number of basic, practical efforts to combat the sustainable agriculture epidemic. There are numerous applications in sustainable agriculture and food systems that are routinely used by working people. Farmers can employ a variety of techniques that utilize less water, increase soil health, and reduce pollution on farms. Consumers and retailers interested in sustainability can seek out food that is produced using practices that encourage farmworker well-being, are environmentally benign or help to develop the local economy [3].

Sustainable agriculture, on the other hand, is more than a set of procedures. Many industrial technologies, such as chemical fertilizers, pesticides, and mechanical equipment, have been incorporated into agriculture production to meet the demand for food. This type of overall operation harms the agricultural sector's land, water, air, and native habitats. The United Nations' Sustainable Development Goals (SDGs), adopted in 2015, emphasize the critical relevance of sustainable agriculture for global development. Sustainable agriculture began with a farming concept that is more environmentally, economically, and socially responsible. The community's research is gradually deepening as sustainable agriculture techniques become more prevalent. Sustainable agricultural development is the focus of nano fertilizers, high-yielding rice, biotechnology, and other emerging technologies [4, 5]. Where food comes from and how it is produced is one of the most critical maintenance issues in the twenty-first century. Every day, as more than 7 billion people live more complex lives, the difficulty of sustaining life in a crowded world grows. As the year progresses, the population continues to rise. Knowing the dilemma, it will be tough to feed everyone. As the population grows, more money will be required for spending.

## EFFECT OF SUSTAINABLE AGRICULTURE

While agriculture activity might help to preserve biodiversity, it can also threaten uncultivated species and space. Agriculture allows for many of the environmental concerns that WWF actively targets, from habitat loss to pollution [6, 7].

*Land modification:* Agriculture spread is a critical cause of deforestation and other ecological degradation, destroying domain and biodiversity. Oil palms, for example, are displacing lowland forests in Indonesia, while soy farming is destroying Brazil's Atlantic forests. Extreme erosion can be seen as a result of forest loss and unsustainable farming practises. Half of all agricultural topsoil has been destroyed in the last 50 years [6-8].

*Pollution:* Agriculture is the main source of pollution in many countries. The use of pesticides, fertilizers, and other toxic chemicals can ruin the freshwater, marine ecosystem, air, and soil. They can also live a long life in the environment. Many pesticides disrupt the hormones which are present in wildlife and humans.

*Scarcity:* Agriculture is the only valuable resource for most of the world's extremely poor people. In many countries, the agriculturalists are forced to encourage over-production, which decreases the prices. Producers face a decrease meant in harvesting from clean land which converts into surrounding wildlands that are rich in biodiversity, resulting in a cycle of increasing poverty.

*Water consumption:* The agriculture industry utilises more than half of all freshwater on the planet. Agriculture production wastes too much water and affects water quality if water is not used properly. This demonstrates the negative impact on the global freshwater system.

*Weather conditions:* Much agricultural work like burning unwanted plants and using gasoline powdered machinery – are the main developer produce greenhouse gases in the surrounding. The food and agriculture organization of the united nation (FAO) conflicts that the life stock sector alone is responsible for 18% of all greenhouse gas production. Furthermore, cleaning solid ground for farming productivity is also a measure helper to weather change, as the carbon present in the absolute forest is released when they are burned or cut [6-10].

## WHAT WFF IS DOING

WFF acknowledges and prefers farmland management operations. We provide economic stimulants to encourage biodiversity preservation, enhance agricultural regulations, and identify new revenue opportunities for farmers. Agriculture techniques that are managed sustainably can assist to maintain and restore vital natural environments, as well as improving soil health and water quality [9-11]. WFF collaborates with a diverse group of individuals to:

- Reduce and define the effect to extend the priority commodities on the stakeholders' roundtables.
- Save the environment and growers' bottom line for the better implementation of management practices.
- Produce economic stimulants to promote biodiversity conservation.
- Improves agricultural policies.
- Point out the new idea to ensure growers' economy.

## BENEFITS OF SUSTAINABLE AGRICULTURE

There are benefits to committing to the advancement of technologically driven agricultural practices so that we can continue to progress toward the benefits of sustainable agriculture [12, 13].

- *Environmental conservation and pollution prevention:* Farmers who adopt sustainable practices reduce their reliance on non-renewable energy, reduce chemical use, conserve exotic resources, and conserve land to save and replenish can go a long way in addressing the growing population and demand for food.
- *Cutting costs and concentrating on profits:* Farming more effectively and moving food straight from the farm will benefit everyone involved in the agriculture industry.
- *Increasing food production without wasting it:* As previously said, population growth is a matter of concern. There are numerous potentials to enhance agriculture techniques from pure production today, and sustainable agriculture is the source of even more possibilities.

## CHALLENGES OF SUSTAINABLE AGRICULTURE

Three agriculture sector challenges will be important to India's overall development and improved welfare [14, 15]:

*Raising agriculture productivity per unit of land:* Water is essential for irrigation to overcome industrial and rural needs, as the source is limited the important part for growth in agriculture and fertilized land per unit productivity must be increased. To decrease marketing expenses we must develop a chain to alter high-value crops and yield progressively, this method insure that fertility is increased.

A socially comprehensive strategy is used to reduce rural poverty that includes cooperation between agriculture and non-farm employment: The poverty-stricken homeless women's, backward caste should profit from the development in rural areas. Furthermore, most of India's poverty-stricken people depend on the weather which creates a strong imbalance in the region. An improvement has been seen in the rural population which was around 40% in the 1990s reduced to 30% in the mid-2000s but it is facing enough as eradication of poverty and development should be the main focus of the government.

*Certification of agricultural progress promotes food security:* In the 1970s, the green revolution increased foodgrain output, allowing the country to become food grain self-sufficient and reduce hunger anxieties. Increased demand for rural labour in the 1970s and 1980s increased rural income, which, along with decreasing food prices, reduced rural poverty. Between the 1990s and the 2000s, agricultural growth slowed, yet cereal yields increased by 1.4 percent each year. Agriculture's slowing growth has been a key source of concern. As a result, policymakers will need to start or finish policy measures and public programmes to move the category away from the existing policy, which appears to be unsustainable, and lay the basis for a considerably more productive, competitive, and diverse agriculture sector.

## MAIN COMPONENTS OF SUSTAINABLE AGRICULTURE

Soil management, crop management, water management, disease/pest management, and waste management are the primary components of sustainable farming. The methods employed are frequently vastly different. Crop rotation and a high amount of compost and green manure, which are plowed crops produced in soil containing organic matter, are used in sustainable agriculture to maintain and improve soil fertility. Sustainable agriculture uses a wide variety of crops and meticulous rotation to ensure that nutrients are replenished naturally and that no single pest or disease gets out of hand [8-11].

In sustainable irrigate management, water is seen as a valuable resource, and it is efficiently managed to water crops by drip irrigation, which causes erosion and evaporation. Farmers in dry climates use efficient water because they plant drought-resistant crops and have fewer animals to graze. In sustainable farming, plants and animals are encouraged to use their natural resistance rather than pesticides. Animals who are allowed to graze freely and eat a healthy diet are less prone to illness and disease. Microbes help plants grow well, and nutrient-rich soil keeps bugs and illnesses at bay. If a pest or disease must be eradicated, sustainable farmers employ natural methods.

## REFERENCES

1. De Olde, E.M., Oudshoorn, F.W., Sørensen, C.A.G., Bokkers, E.A.M., De Boer, I.J.M. Assessing Sustainability at Farm-level: Lessons Learned from a Comparison of Tools in Practice. Ecol Indic 2016; 66: 391-404.
2. Slätmo, E., Fischer, K. and Roos, E. The Framing of Sustainability in Sustainability Assessment Frameworks for Agriculture. Sociol Rural 2017; 57: 378-395.
3. Deytieux, V., Munier-Jolain, N. and Caneill, J. Assessing the Sustainability of Cropping Systems in Single- and Multi-site Studies. A Review of methods. Eur J Agron 2016; 72: 107-126.
4. Kropff, M.J., Bouma, J. and Jones, J.W. Systems approaches for the Design of Sustainable Agro-ecosystems. Agric Syst 2001; 70: 369-393.
5. Gold, M.V. (Ed.) Sustainable Agriculture: Definitions and Terms. In Sustainable Agriculture and Food Supply. Apple Academic Press: Waretown NJ USA 2016.
6. Dahlberg, K.A. Sustainable Agriculture: Fad or Harbinger? BioScience 1991; 41: 337-340.

7. Darnhofer, I., Bellon, S., Dedieu, B. and Milestad, R. Adaptiveness to Enhance the Sustainability of Farming Systems. A review. Agron Sustain Dev 2010; 30: 545-555.
8. Hill, S.B. and MacRae, R.J. Conceptual Framework for the Transition from Conventional to Sustainable Agriculture. J Sustain Agric 1996; 7: 81-87.
9. Le Gal, P.Y., Merot, A., Moulin, C.H., Navarrete, M. and Wery, J. A modelling Framework to Support Farmers in Designing Agricultural Production Systems. Environ Model Softw 2010; 25: 258-268.
10. Gomez-Limon, J.A. and Sanchez-Fernandez, G. Empirical Evaluation of Agricultural Sustainability using Composite Indicators. Ecol Econ 2010; 69: 1062-1075.
11. Acosta-Alba, I. and Van der Werf, H. The Use of Reference Values in Indicator-Based methods for the Environmental Assessment of Agricultural Systems. Sustainability 2011; 3: 424-442.
12. Carof, M., Colomb, B. and Aveline, A. A Guide for Choosing the most Appropriate method for Multi-criteria Assessment of Agricultural Systems according to Decision-makers' Expectations. Agric Syst 2013; 115: 51-62.
13. Schader, C., Grenz, J., Meier, M.S. and Stolze, M. Scope and Precision of Sustainability Assessment Approaches to Food Systems. Ecol Soc 2014; 19.
14. Schiefer, J., Lair, G.J. and Blum, W.E.H. Indicators for the definition of Land Quality as a basis for the Sustainable Intensification of Agricultural Production. Int. Soil Water Conserv Res 2015; 3: 42-49.
15. Repar, N., Jan, P., Dux, D., Nemecek, T. and Doluschitz, R. Implementing Farm-level Environmental Sustainability in Environmental performance Indicators: A Combined Global-local Approach. J Clean Prod 2017; 140: 692-704.

**Corresponding author: Dr. Amit Gupta, Associate Professor, Department of Biotechnology, Graphic Era (Deemed to be) University, Dehradun, India.**
**Email id: dr.amitgupta.bt@geu.ac.in**

Pages: 94-100
**Emerging Environmental Contaminants and Global Healthcare Systems**
*Editors:* **Prof. (Dr.) Shyam Narain Pandey; Murtaza Abid**
**Prof. (Dr.) Syed Rais Haider; Dr. Sabiha Kazmi; Dr. Mohd. Zahid Rizvi**
*ISBN:* **978-81-959169-2-4**
*Edition:* **2023**
*Published by:* **Discovery Publishing House, New Delhi (India)**

# Conception of Urban Ecology

**Smriti Khare, Amit Gupta**

**ABSTRACT**

*Across all three dimensions of sustainable development, urban ecology is a cross-cutting issue. Economic reasons drive urbanization in developing countries while large ecological footprints allow developed countries to reduce their environmental impact through efficient urban planning. Urbanization has led to a more domesticated environment worldwide. Urban ecosystem services and human well-being have become a top focus of research activities in the field as it emerges as a paradigm for urban sustainability. In terms of the interaction of humans and their natural environments, urban areas are a test-bed and living lab. In general, urban growth pattern is more familiar in terms of space and time which may understand the mechanism and factors of urbanization including myriad ecological effects. In short, development of sustainability and urban ecology are key factors for transitioning to a sustainable world.*

***Keywords:*** *sustainable; urbanization; ecosystem and ecology.*

## INTRODUCTION

An urban ecology is a multidisciplinary field that examines the interrelationships between living organisms (including humans) and their nonliving (abiotic) environments within an urban setting. In Darwinian terms, ecology is defined as the science of studying interactions between organisms and their environment, as well as their consequences at all spatial and temporal scales. Ecologists refer to biodiversity as a key concept because

**Department of Life Sciences and Biotechnology, Graphic Era Deemed to be University, Dehradun (India)**

it captures the diversity of life at all scales: genes, species, ecosystems. In accordance with our definition, the Carry Institute of Ecosystem Studies focuses on the holistic and encompassing perspective of ecology, as 'the scientific study of processes influencing the distribution and abundance of organisms, the interactions among organisms, and the transformation and flux of energy and matter.' This field of study integrates the theory and methods of both natural and social sciences to study the patterns and processes of urban ecosystems, hence encompasses many disciplines; geography, ecology, sociology, architecture, planning, and human health, to name just a few. Ecological planning also an endeavour that is fundamentally practical [1, 2]. Inspite of the fact that the urbanized land community or neighbourhood governed by the built or assembled environment – "all non-vegetative, human-constructed elements, such as buildings, roads, runways, etc." – inhabited small percentage of the earth's terrestrial surface, consequence of urbanization are intense and prevalent from the local to the global scale. In normal survey, where cities mainly accounted residential water use (60%), energy use (75%), wood (80% for industrial purposes) and greenhouse emissions through human (80%). As urbanization has increased, a variety of new forms of urban development have emerged over the last 50 years. As a result, ecosystems, landscapes, and even biosphere, have been greatly domesticated, hastening the arrival of the Anthropocene era [1-4].

## CHARACTERISTICS OF AN URBAN AREA

McIntyre *et al.* (2000) argue for the integration of social and natural science and fully understand the term to enable interproject comparability and replicability of findings. There are three major factors used to define urban areas i.e. population (total size, density, and surface area or assembled structures). In general, these urban areas will have incorporated some common features: high population density, plentiful built structures, extensive impervious surfaces, altered climatic and hydrological conditions, air pollution, and modified ecosystem function and services [5, 6].

## URBAN ECOSYSTEM: EFFECTS, PROS & CONS

Natural ecosystems are changed tremendously by urbanization in countless biological, hydrologic, and even geomorphic ways. The urbanization of places results in the filling of wetlands, razing of woodlands, flattening of hillsides, and the severance of migration routes. Plants and animals can become isolated within fragmented land uses as a result of fragmented land use patterns, which could eventually lead to their extirpation. Animals moving from one habitat patch to another are threatened by collisions with vehicles, attacks (from dogs, for example), predation, and disease. Suburbanization in many parts of Australia, for instance, is now threatening the koalas (e.g., tree thinning). In cities, temperature, water levels, nutrients and soil acidity fluxes are radically altered, resulting in major changes in hydrological and biogeochemical cycles. All of these factors can alter the distribution and composition of species found in these locations, perhaps leading to the emergence of new ecologies.

Urbanization and changes to coastal processes have profound effects on coastal areas and coastlines. Coastal areas and near-shore groundwater can be affected by septic system leaks due to drawdown from coastal aquifers. The coastal marine environment near the shore can be significantly polluted and polluted by highly urbanized rivers. As a result of these changes urban residents, plants, and animals may be susceptible to flooding, coastal erosion and landslides [5-8]. In fact, rats, pigeons, and sparrows exist in harmony with humans in the urban matrices - and thrive there. As a result of urbanization, nonindigenous species are introduced into urban habitats (deliberately or accidentally). The most important threat to biodiversity today is invasive non-native species, followed by habitat loss. Urbanization prompts adaptive responses. Plants and animals must be able to exchange genes in order for urban wildlife to flourish. Breeding cycles, interactions' duration and predictability, and seasonality are factors that affect an area's seasonality. In areas where species persist, changes in behaviour will occur. Eventually, breeding patterns, spawning, breeding patterns and the nature of individual organisms can all be altered as a result of these impacts. There has been evidence that some birds and frogs modify their pitches and/or the frequencies of their calls in urban areas to prevent their calls from being drowned out by ambient urban noise.

Both positive and negative effects of urban habitats and wildlife can be observed on humans. Animal attacks on people and pets are a few negative effects; related to disease spread (e.g., Lyme disease); physical damage to houses caused by nesting; physical damage to gardens caused by insect attack, animal foraging, and/or trampling; and loud vocalizations (e.g., the North American mockingbird, which calls at night). Property damage can be caused by urban trees, as well as preventing the flow of light, causing allergies and asthma, and attracting nuisance wildlife.

However, urban residents can also benefit from access to urban nature. These benefits include economic advantages, recreational benefits, and environmental benefits. Pollution abatement, noise attenuation, and carbon sequestration are all ecosystem services. It has aesthetic value, spiritual value, provides stress relief, and promotes socialization [5-8].

## EVOLVING URBAN LANDSCAPES: DECADES OF CHANGE

The following sections summarize the major advances on several research fronts i.e.

## Spatiotemporal Patterns of Urbanization

Urban space patterns include a variety of factors, such as distribution of green spaces, waterways, transportation networks, and patterns of urban growth. The study of urban growth patterns has progressed in two ways over the past decades. Thanks to continuous improvements in remote sensing and GIS techniques, we can now analyse urbanization patterns at multiple spatial and temporal scales, from cities to the entire globe. The amalgam of theoretical development along with studies related to empirical which may have resulted in a more broadly way and understanding the concept of urban growth form.

Geographical variation in urban landscapes is related to a variety of physical environments, socioeconomic factors, and land use policies. Landscape ecology may help pertaining to resolve these multiplex issues. As remote sensing, geographic information systems, and spatial analysis have evolved, so have our tools for analysing the spatiotemporal patterns of urbanization [9-11].

## Urban Biodiversity and Environment Processes

Since the 1970s, studies of urban ecology and environment have fascinated primarily on determining the impacts of urbanization on biodiversity and ecological condition. Depending on taxonomic groups, environmental conditions, and socioeconomics, urbanization affects biodiversity differently. Scientists at the CAP-LTER report a declining in predation pressure on birds allowed certain species of avian species to flourish, and avian predators were more effective at controlling arthropod herbivores in urban environments than in rural ones [9-12].

Landscape homogenization tends to reduce habitat heterogeneity for biological species, suggesting that urbanization explains biotic homogeneity. Human activities in urban environments have also been documented to cause an array of environmental problems, including greenhouse gas emissions, solid waste and air and water pollution. By increasing water use, contaminating water, altering runoff patterns, and changing evapotranspiration rates, urbanization influences hydrological cycling and stream flow patterns in urban areas. Aside from climate change, urbanization also affects the timing and duration of vegetation phenology, or landscape phenology - the timing and duration of a plant's development phase triggered by environmental factors. UHIs have the potential to alter both the timing and duration of plant growth and blooming as a result of changing temperature and moisture conditions [10-13].

## Urbanization and Human Well-Being

Biological diversity and ecosystem function (or process) makes up natural capital stock, the stock of natural resources that humans rely on for goods and services. The Millennium Ecosystem Assessment, 2005 defined ecosystem services as "the benefits people obtain from ecosystems" which provides a number of services that includes, provisioning industry (such as food and water), synchronize services (i.e. flooding, disease control, hazard control, and noise control), cultural practices (i.e. recreation, spirituality, and religious experience) and supporting services (i.e. soil formation, primary production, and nutrient cycling) [12-14].

As per the study of Bolund and Hunhammar, identified seven types of local ecosystems (i.e. street trees, parks, urban forests, cultivated land, wetlands, lakes and sea, and streams). These ecosystem services led to significant improvements in the quality of life for local residents, including air filtration, heat regulation, noise reduction, rainwater drainage, sewage treatment, recreation, and cultural activities.

Studies of urban landscape patterns and their effects on human and social well-being have mostly relied on correlational analysis; the causes and mechanisms behind these effects are yet to be explored deeply. Research findings and methods from several fields are needed to improve this situation, including cultural geographies, environmental psychology, sociology, landscape ecology, and urban planning and design [13-15].

**Urban Sustainability, Indicators and Integrated Approach**

Those urban ecologies that meet ethical, effective (healthy and equitable), zero-waste generation, self-regulation, resilience, self-renewal, flexibility, psychological fulfilment, and cooperative requirements are sustainable. In today's world, cities are considered an important laboratory for human-environment interactions and urbanization is considered a global experiment in sustainability. Although we cannot predict the outcome of the experiment, we do know its significance: it will determine the fate of humankind. Sustainable development, therefore, must be incorporated into urban ecology's scientific foundation and be its overarching goal. It has already begun, but there is still much more to be done [15-17].

Any system's progress can be assessed using indicators. A number of aspects of urban systems are considered in terms of urban sustainability indicators, including policy and governance, demographics, economics, environment and energy. There are several types of indicators, such as gross domestic product, Gini coefficient, and ambient air quality. By using indicators, we can gain insight into the phenomenon we are studying.

Human beings now primarily live in urban areas. Whether urban ecology occurs "in" or "of" the city, it remains fundamental to the planned, designed, and managed built environment in the 21st century, from the room to the region. Professionals in the built environment need to have a practical knowledge of ecologies and their application in our rapidly urbanizing world, as well as an understanding of the importance of urban ecosystem services. These findings will not only aid in tackling the defining challenge of our time, climate change, but will also contribute to maintaining and enhancing the resilience, liability, and health of our urban spaces, as well as to ensuring the wellbeing of their inhabitants [16, 17].

## CONCLUSION

Many problems were facing today i.e. biodiversity loss, air pollution, lack of green space, and a lack of open space. In the long term, though, there is evidence that cities are resilient ecosystems, which is why their performance continues to improve. It would be helpful to create a sustainable future with policies informed by an understanding of how urban ecosystems work. In light of the urbanization phenomenon across the globe, the study of the urban ecosystem has been given increasing spotlight to ensure sustainability of resource use. The importance of environmental conservation in urban ecology cannot be overstated. As most of the world's population has been moving to cities, urban ecology has become increasingly important. Global urban sprawl has the consequence that cities are expanding into environmentally sensitive regions, where pollution and land conversion of natural habitats alter ecosystem structure. The knowledge gained from studying biological communities in cities may assist established cities as the planet continues to urbanize. Research into urban ecology is crucial to understanding planet-wide ecosystem dynamics. Biodiversity is a key element of a successful urban ecosystem, and humans get to experience the benefits of urban ecosystems by having access to nature. We can work together in order to keep a diversity of species even in cities. In this way, we can have a better future with less environmental destruction.

## REFERENCES

1. Grimm, N.B., Faeth, S.H., Golubiewski, N.E., Redman, C.L., Wu, J., Bai, X., *et al.* Global Change and the Ecology of Cities. Science 2008; 319: 756-760.
2. McIntyre, N.E., Knowles-Yanez, K. and Hope, D. Urban Ecology as an Interdisciplinary Field: Differences in the use of 'Urban' between the Social and Natural Sciences. Urban Ecosystems 2000; 4 (1): 5-24.
3. Newman, P., Beatley, T. and Boyer, H. Resilient Cities: Responding to Peak Oil and Climate change. Washington, DC: Island Press. Global Change and the Ecology of Cities. Science 2009; 319 (5864): 756-760.
4. Paul, O. and Natalie, P. Urban Ecology as an Interdisciplinary Area, Encyclopaedia of Sustainable Technologies Elsevier 2017; 31-42.
5. McKinney, M.L. Urbanization as a Major cause of Biotic Homogenization. Biological Conservation 2006; 127: 247-260.
6. Pickett, S.T.A., Cadenasso, M.L., Grove, J.M., Nilon, C.H., Pouyat, R.V., Zipperer, W.C., *et al.* Urban Ecological Systems: Linking Terrestrial Ecological, Physical, and Socioeconomic Components of Metropolitan Areas. Annual Review of Ecology Evolution and Systematics 2001; 32: 127-157.

7. Marzluff, J. and Rodewald, A. Conserving Biodiversity in Urbanizing Areas: Non-traditional views from a Bird's Perspective. Cities and the Environment (CATE) 2008; 1 (2): 6.
8. De Groot, R.S., Wilson, M.A. and Boumans, R.M.J. A Typology for the Classification, Description and Valuation of Ecosystem Functions, Goods and Services. Ecological Economics 2002; 41: 393-408.
9. Batty, M. Agents, Cells, and Cities: New Representational models for Simulating Multiscale Urban Dynamics. Environment and Planning A 2005; 37: 1373-1394.
10. Batty, M. and Longley, P. Urban Growth and form: Scaling, Fractal Geometry, and Diffusion-limited Aggregation. Environment and Planning A 1989; 21: 1447-1472.
11. Herold, M., Goldstein, N.C. and Clarke, K.C. The Spatiotemporal form of Urban Growth: Measurement, Analysis and Modelling. Remote Sensing of Environment 2003; 86: 286-302.
12. Faeth, S.H., Warren, P.S., Shochat, E. and Marussich, W.A. Trophic Dynamics in Urban Communities. BioScience 2005; 55: 399-407.
13. Neil, K. and Wu, J. Effects of Urbanization on Plant Flowering Phenology. Urban Ecosystems 2006; 9: 243-257.
14. Neil K, Landrum L, Wu JG. Effects of Urbanization on Flowering Phenology in the Metropolitan Region of USA: Findings from Herbarium Records. Journal of Arid Environments 2010; 74: 440-444.
15. Schaich H, Bieling C, Plieninger T. Linking Ecosystem Services with Cultural Landscape Research. GAIA 2010; 19: 269-277.
16. Verma P, Raghubanshi AS. Urban Sustainability Indicators: Challenges and Opportunities. Ecological Indicators 2018; 93: 282e291.
17. Dizdaroglu D. Developing Micro-level Urban Ecosystem Indicators for Sustainability Assessment. Environmental Impact Assessment Review 2015; 54: 119-124.

**Corresponding author: Dr Amit Gupta, Associate Professor, Department of Biotechnology, Graphic Era (Deemed to be) University, Dehradun, India.**
**Email id: dr.amitgupta.bt@geu.ac.in**

Pages: 101-109

**Emerging Environmental Contaminants and Global Healthcare Systems**

*Editors:* **Prof. (Dr.) Shyam Narain Pandey; Murtaza Abid**
**Prof. (Dr.) Syed Rais Haider; Dr. Sabiha Kazmi; Dr. Mohd. Zahid Rizvi**

*ISBN:* **978-81-959169-2-4**

*Edition:* **2023**

*Published by:* **Discovery Publishing House, New Delhi (India)**

# Contaminants in the Environment
## *Water Pollution*

**Lovy Singh Bist, Karneshwar Gholia**
**Mrityunjay Mishra, Amit Gupta**

### ABSTRACT

*Human activities and the rapid rise in population is the major cause behind the introduction of pollutants and hazardous substances in water making it contaminated which has led to the "loss of vigour of water bodies" along with the eradication of ecosystem causing many environmental problems and also causing to widespread of water borne diseases. These water borne diseases may be due to chemicals which directly contaminate our land, water and soil. In other words, these chemicals may directly or indirectly contaminate the water which may affect the environment including human health. In addition, water containing chemicals also effect on large coastal areas and threatening human health. This chapter tries to discuss what water pollution is along with its sources, effects, control measures and management.*

***Keywords:*** *Contaminants; water; pollution and management.*

## INTRODUCTION

Water is the driving force of nature. There is no life on this earth without water and hence its importance is to be greatly emphasized. Water is important for all living being inhabits this earth, be it plant, animal and all human beings. Plants need water to carry out the process of photosynthesis and to provide them with nutrients essential for their

**Department of Biotechnology, Graphic Era (Deemed to be) University, Dehradun, (India)**

growths through the process of active and passive transport. The 60% of body weight of human and animals comprises of water. The cells, organs and tissues require water for maintaining homeostasis and carrying out different metabolic process. We also require water for domestic purposes like cooking food, cleaning, washing clothes and also for irrigation and cultivation of crops. Water is also needed in industries to carry out different processes. The total volume on earth is estimated to be 1.3896-billion-kilometer cube, with 97.5% being salt water and 2.5 % being fresh water and of which only 0.3% is in liquid form on the surface (i.e. for consumption). So, the depletion of this commodity either through contamination or careless use can result in serious consequences. Hence, the importance of water for the substance of life cannot be overemphasized and so proper measures need to be taken for the preventing water pollution at all levels with an initiative to protect and preserve our water bodies [1, 2].

Olaniran (1995) defined water pollution to be the presence of excessive amount of a hazard (pollutant) in water in such a way that it is no long suitable for drinking, bathing, cooking, or other uses. Water is known as the universal solvent as it can dissolve more substances than any other liquid on this earth, making it uniquely vulnerable. Toxic substances from households, farms, towns, industries and factories when introduced into water bodies like (streams, rivers, lakes, etc.) readily dissolve into and mix with it causing water pollution. According to a recent survey on national quality from (U.S. Environmental Protection Agency) "nearly half of our rivers and lakes are polluted." Making them unfit for carrying out essential activities like drinking, irrigation, cultivation, fishing, etc. The toxic substance in contaminated water causes severe water borne diseases and also disturbs the natural flora and fauna of the water bodies [3-5]. The wide spread problem of water pollution is jeopardizing our health and so serious measures need to be taken for making water pollution free.

## SOURCES OF WATER POLLUTION

Humans achieve more advancement in technology and science century after century, but at the cost of the degradation of our environment. Mankind is responsible for introducing pollutants into water bodies. The rise in human population, rapid industrialization, overcrowding of urban areas and increase in agricultural practices are some major causes of pollution. The following are some major causes behind the pollution of water.

- **Agricultural Waste (Fertilizers and Pesticides):** The food demand has risen intensively with the rapid growth of population leading to the increase in areas equipped for irrigation purposes. Current times need a greater yield of crop hence the use of different fertilizers and pesticides has increased. These are not fully consumed by the crops and are washed off with the top layer of the soil during rain and enter into nearby streams. They contain chemicals like nitrogen, phosphorus, sulphur, etc. which enables algae to grow at a faster rate and cause acute health effects [6].

- **Industrial Waste:** The emergence of various industries coupled with the development of civilization has constantly increased the quantity of waste water containing pollutants. Metal mining industries, textile and leather factories, sugar mills, petroleum industries and many others are held responsible for polluting water bodies. The waste products from these industries include suspended solids of high concentration along with metal ions and hazardous chemicals like sulphuric acid, when discharged into water bodies directly exert large influence on the natural environment [7].
- **Oil Spills:** Oil is denser than water and does not dissolve in it, forms a thick sludge. Thousands of oil spills happen accidently each year, maybe small for example if oil spills while refuelling a ship or they can be a major disaster if the oil spills due to pipelines breaks, ships with big oil tankers sink or when the drilling operation goes wrong. It takes a large amount of time and effort to remove the layer of oil accumulated over the surface of water. These spills cause major damage to the ecosystem and the marine life inhabiting the site especially if they happen in sensitive environment, the consequences of which can be felt for decades [8].
- **Untreated Sewage:** Sewage is the liquid waste containing solid organic matter and a mixture of human faeces along with waste water from other household activities. This sewage is the biggest cause behind water pollution. The untreated sewage contains many disease-causing pathogens and other toxic materials; hence sewage should be treated properly in sewage treatment plants before being discharged into waterbodies [9].

Other activities like littering in public places, improper waste disposal, leaked sewer lines, dumping of household waste, increased urbanization and industrialization etc., also cause water pollution. Hence mankind as a whole is responsible for polluting water through activities carried on to better self-growth.

## EFFECT OF WATER POLLUTION

Water pollution, in today's times, is a major problem that requires urgent and permanent treatment. Waste from industries, households, dumping of harming waste chemicals and hazardous medical waste are causing deterioration of the water quality and also increases the water toxicity. Due to this, the level of available drinkable water has decreased significantly in these past few years. It has also destroyed many aquatic life forms.

- **On Aquatic Life:** The recent upsurge in water pollution has caused severe damage to the aquatic ecosystem. The aquatic ecosystem mainly suffers because of the dropping level of fresh oxygenated water. The organic waste material escalates the BOD (Biological Oxygen Demand) as a lot of bacteria and microorganisms are required to decompose all that matter under aerobic conditions. All the inorganic waste, which can't get dissolved in water on its own/naturally, releases many harmful toxins in water like potassium, calcium, sodium, magnesium, sulphate, chloride, nitrate, etc. All these inorganic and organic water pollutants raise the toxicity of water, which makes it unfit for many living organisms and, due to which, many life forms are dead or their number is significantly low. This in turn disturbs the food chain, which is also causing damage to many other spices [10].
- **On Human's health:** Consumption or the usage of polluted water can bring about health issues, including digestive issues, toxicity and loss of life, or chronic toxicity and neurological problems from extra critical chemical pollutants. Polluted water contains a lot of harmful waterborne pathogens which can cause a lot of major diseases in humans. In the majority of people, Giardia, typhoid, and cholera are caused by this polluted water. In some places, water pollution is also caused by accidental breakage or illegal opening of sewerage pipelines. Water contaminated by sewerage contains faecal contaminants, which are very hazardous for humans and also contains bacteria responsible for diseases like diarrhoea, cholera, polio, hepatitis A, and dysentery. Polluted water contains microplastics in abundance. Humans' digestive system is unable to break or pass out microplastics. So, this microplastic gets stuck in the human body for several years and can cause inflammatory reactions and metabolic disorders. Ingestion of chemical pollutants like fertilizers, chemical waste, pesticides, and heavy metals causes health risks. If consumed regularly or for a long time, it can also cause cancer, hormone disruption, altered brain function, damage to immune and reproductive systems, and cardiovascular and kidney problems. Consumption is not the only way in which polluted water can cause harm to humans' body. The contaminated water can also come in contact with our skin in many day-to-day routines, like while swimming or while washing clothes. Polluted water after coming in contact with human skin can cause rashes, eye reddening, skin cancer and severe skin irritation [11, 12].

## CONTROL AND MANAGEMENT OF WATER POLLUTION

Water pollution is a major concern, as it affects the life of both flora and fauna, but there are some methods through which water pollution can be controlled [13-18].

- *Reducing the use of plastic:* Plastic substances have toxic chemical elements like chlorine, which can cause harmful effects on the health of species drinking that water and as they are non-biodegradable, when they are dumped into the water bodies, they stay for a longer period of time and can cause a lot of problems for the aquatic life. Usage of plastic material that can be further reused must be done.
- *Recycling of waste material:* Substances that can be easily recycled should be used. There are some substances that can be recycled such as tires, metal, paper, plastic etc. Due to which, the contamination of water bodies can be controlled.
- *Proper decomposition of medical waste:* The improper disposal of biomedical waste make calls false impact on the water quality as medical wastes contain microorganisms which have harmful effects, for example: toxic substances from medical waste dumped in water bodies affects the aquatic life and organisms who have absorbed such wastes. search medical waste are then passed along with the food chain which can affect everything from producer to tertiary consumer. Decontamination of medical waste can be done by thermal processing and medical shredders.
- *Limiting the use of fertilizers and pesticides:* Fertilizers and pesticides are composed of some substances such as phosphorus, nitrogen and some unwanted toxic substances which contaminates marine bodies and affect the organisms present in it. When the toxins present in fertilizers and pesticides are exposed in water bodies, the nutritive value of water increases which leads to the growth of algae. This enrichment leads to the depletion of oxygen dissolved in the water bodies. This phenomenon is also known as Eutrophication. Hence, the use of fertilisers should be limited. Besides this, the usage of manures and plantation of nitrogen fixer crops should be increased.
- *Using environment friendly products:* Products made up of bamboo, jute, paper, wood etc must be used as they are biodegradable in nature and can help in controlling water pollution to a greater extent.
- *Proper dumping of industrial waste:* Industries such as radioactive power plant flushes out large amount of toxic waste in water bodies which contains heavy and harmful material search as lead which affects the aquatic life.
- *Use of phosphate free detergents:* Phosphates can cause a variety of water pollution problems as they Do not biodegrade completely and they contaminate our water supplies.
- *Plantation of trees:* Trees reduce erosion that washes pollution into the water. Erosion is the wearing a way of materials found in soil through some external forces like wind and water.

Apart from these methods, there are some techniques which can help in the treatment of polluted water.

- *Sewage water treatment:* The process of cleaning or eliminating the pollutants, treating wastewater and making it safe and suitable for drinking purposes is termed as sewage water treatment. It aims to remove contaminants from wastewater. The process is subdivided into three parts or processes:

**Primary or Physical Treatment:** This is a physical process that involves the processes of sedimentation and sequential filtration to remove the solid debris (large/small) from the sewage. The sewage is firstly mixed with water and diluted, shredded and churned. It is then moved to the filtration tank to remove large floating objects. The filtered sewage is passed into a gravity settlement tank where coarse particles (like sand, pebbles, stones) settle down. After this the sewage is passed into a "primary settling tank" with a gentle slope. The sewage is then passed forward for secondary treatment. The solid material along with organic matter that is screened out during the primary treatment is called the "primary sludge". This primary sludge constitutes of organic matter that can be directly or indirectly used for the production of biogas and compost or manure.

**Secondary or Biological Treatment:** There are many methods for performing secondary treatment, such as oxidation tank and trickling filer, but the most commonly used method is Activated sludge method. The secondary treatment is a biological process which makes use of the degrading activities of microbes for digestion of organic matter. The primary effluent is passed into an aeration tank and a certain amount of inoculum (activated sludge from previous cycle) is added into it to allow the growth of aerobic microbes. In this tank air is pumped continuously and is constantly agitated mechanically. This leads to the growth of many aerobic microbes in the aeration tank which include filamentous fungi, algae, protozoa, and bacteria. These microbes form masses appearing in the form of mesh like structures which are called "flocs". The growth of these microbes' results in the digestion of the major part of the organic matter of the effluent. This results in considerable amount of the BOD (Biological oxygen demand) of the effluent. The sewage water is treated till the entire BOD is reduced. The BOD is a measure of the level of contamination (amount of different origin matter) present in water so the greater is the BOD of waste water, the greater is its polluting potential. Now, the microbial flocs in the sewage are allowed to settle down into a sedimentation tank. The substance that settles down after the secondary treatment has been carried out is called the "activated sludge."

**Tertiary treatment:** A small amount of this activated sludge is pumped back into the aeration tank as an inoculum; the remaining part is pumped into a "aerobic sludge digester" tank. An oxygen free environment is maintained in this tank, where anaerobic microorganisms start digesting the bacteria and fungi in the sludge. The effluent now is considerably very less of BOD and hence can be released into water bodies. While the anaerobic microorganisms carry out the anaerobic digestion, they produce a mixture of gasses (methane, carbon-di-oxide, hydrogen sulphide) which is highly inflammable. While the spent sludge can be used as a compost or manure in farms.

- *Reverse osmosis:* This method helps in the removal of contaminants from water by using high pressure. During this process, the toxic substances are filtered out and flushed away leaving clean, drinkable water. This process involves the usage of semi permeable or partially permeable membrane which helps in the separation of unwanted molecules and large particles from drinking water. Reverse osmosis is generally used in treating surface and groundwater. Besides this, it is also used in the manufacturing of food, soda, beverages etc.
- *Ion exchange method:* It is a method in which one or more unwanted ionic contaminants are separated from water by exchanging or replacing it with a non-toxic ionic substance.
- *Coagulation:* This method involves the addition of coagulants such as Iron and aluminium salts that have a positive charge which neutralises the negative charge of the particles dissolved in the water. Coagulation removes many unwanted particles which are not required such as organic carbon.

## CASE STUDY OF "RIVER GANGA"

River Ganga, which is worshipped as goddess 'Ganga' by the Hindus, is the lifeline of northern India. Rising in the western Himalayas, this sacred river has a stretch of 2,525 km. It flows through many cities and towns which results in dumping of huge amounts of untreated waste into it. At the same time sewage, industrial waste, idles, half-burnt dead bodies and animal carcass also add to the pollution of water. Most of the times this waste is toxic and non-biodegradable which worsens the situation. This polluted water results in deaths due to water-borne diseases. The World Bank estimates that the health costs of water pollution equal three percent of India's total GDP. It has also suggested that eighty percent of all illness and one-third of deaths in the country are due to water-borne diseases.

## CASE STUDY OF "THE ENVIRONMENTAL POLLUTION OF KANDY LAKE, SRI LANKA"

The water pollution levels of Kandy Lake in Sri Lanka were monitored to probe the impacts and influences of urban environment in a developing country. Although Kandy Lake is a source of drinking water for the town, it was observed that a large number of effluent channels drained into it, carrying a continuous flow of contaminated water. A high coliform count and a high degree of faecal contamination was observed in all water samples obtained from the lake and drains. The pH of water remained almost neutral and provided ideal conditions for bacterial growth. All laboratory and field experiments indicated eutrophic conditions in the lake and the unsuitability of water in the impurified state drinking purposes. Purified water had a zero-coliform value, but the added chlorine content was relatively high and may indicate health risks. Overall, the polluted water in Kandy Lake indicated the adversities of human involvements with nature and provided a good case study for human influence on water pollution in a developing country.

## REFERENCES

1. Lee, B. and Scholz, M. What is the Role of *Phragmites Australis* in Experimental Constructed Wetland Filters Treating Urban runoff? Ecological Engineering 2007; 29: 87-95.
2. Lu, Q., Zhenli, L.H., Graetz, D.A., Stoffella, P.J. and Yang, X. Phytoremediation to remove Nutrients and Improve Eutrophic Storm Waters using Water Lettuce (*Pistia stratiotes* L.). Environmental Science and Pollution Research 2010; 17: 84-96.
3. Miao, Y., Xi-yuan, X., Xu-feng, M., Zhao-hui, G. and Feng-yong, W. Effect of Amendments on Growth and Metal uptake of Giant Reed (*Arundo donax* L.) Grown on Soil Contaminated by Arsenic, Cadmium and Lead. Transactions on Nonferrous Metals Society of China. 2012; 22: 1462-1469.
4. Duffus, J. Heavy Metals - A meaningless Term. Pure and Applied Chemistry 2002; 74(5): 793-807.
5. Blaylock, M.J. and Huang, J.W. In: Raskin I, Ensley BD, Editors. Phytoremediation of Toxic Metals: Using Plants to Clean up the Environment. New York: John Wiley and Sons Inc.; 2000; 53.
6. Adams, B. and Foster, S.S.D. Land-surface Zoning for Groundwater Protection. Water Environ J 1992; 6: 312-319.
7. Chowdhury, S. Exposure Assessment for Trihalomethanes in Municipal Drinking Water and Risk Reduction Strategy. Sci. Total Environ 2013; 463: 922-930.
8. Gunten, U. Ozonation of Drinking Water: Part II. Disinfection and by-product formation in Presence of Bromide, Iodide or Chlorine. Water Res 2003; 37: 1469-1487.
9. Unc, A. and Goss, M.J. Movement of Faecal Bacteria through the Vadose Zone. Water Air Soil Pollut 2003; 149: 327-337.
10. Brodin, T., Piovano, S., Fick, J., Klaminder, J., Heynen, M. and Jonsson, M. Ecological Effects of Pharmaceuticals in Aquatic Systems Impacts through Behavioural Alterations. Philosophical Transactions of the Royal Society B 2014; 369: 20130580.
11. Briggs, D. Environmental Pollution and the Global Burden of Disease. British Medical Bulletin 2003; 68: 1-24.
12. Capkin, E., Allinok, I. and Karahan, S. Water Quality and Fish Size affect Toxicity of Endosulfan an Organochlorine Pesticide to Rainbow Trout. Chemosphere 2006; 64: 1793-1800.

13. Ponsonby, A.L., Couper, D., Dwyer, T., Carmichael, A., Kemp, A. and Cochrane, J. The Relation between Infant Indoor Environment and Subsequent Asthma. Epidemiology 2000; 11: 128-35.

14. Kazan-Allen, L. The Asbestos War. International Journal of Occupational and Environmental Health. 2004; 9: 173-93.

15. Frost, F.J., Tollestrup, K., Craun, G.F., Raucher, R., Chwirka, J. and Stomp, J. Evaluation of Costs and Benefits of Lower Arsenic MCL. Journal AWWA (American Water Works Association). 2002; 94(3): 71-82.

16. Dhara, V.R. and Dhara, R. The Union Carbide Disaster in Bhopal: A Review of Health Effects. Archives of Environmental Health 2002; 57(5): 391-404.

17. Brauer, M. and Hisham-Hashim, J. Indonesian Fires: Crisis and Reaction. Environmental Science and Technology 1998; 32: 404A-7A.

18. Vorosmarty, C.J., Green, P., Salisbury, J. and Lammers, R.B. Global Water Resources: Vulnerability from Climate Change and Population Growth. *Science* 2000; 289: 283-88.

**Corresponding author: Dr Amit Gupta, Associate Professor, Department of Biotechnology, Graphic Era (Deemed to be) University, Dehradun, India.**
**Email id: dr.amitgupta.bt@geu.ac.in**

Pages: 110-124
Emerging Environmental Contaminants and Global Healthcare Systems
*Editors:* Prof. (Dr.) Shyam Narain Pandey; Murtaza Abid
Prof. (Dr.) Syed Rais Haider; Dr. Sabiha Kazmi; Dr. Mohd. Zahid Rizvi
*ISBN:* 978-81-959169-2-4
*Edition:* 2023
*Published by:* Discovery Publishing House, New Delhi (India)

# Ecology and Environmental Contaminants
## *Challenges and Way Forward*

Sri Bharti, Shambhavi Jaiswal, *Pragya Sharma, **Murtaza Abid
***M.M. Abid Ali Khan, V.P. Sharma

## ABSTRACT

*Ecology is an inter-disciplinary science with an improved understanding of urban, peri-urban, and rural complexities with interacting components. Our ecosystem, the earth, essentially controls our economy because it provides us with the resources we require for our economies to function. Resources, materials, and energy are required for long-term human evolution. Furthermore, living organisms influence one another through competition, predation, and other interactions. Ecologists have a better understanding of life processes, adaptations, habitats and biodiversity.*

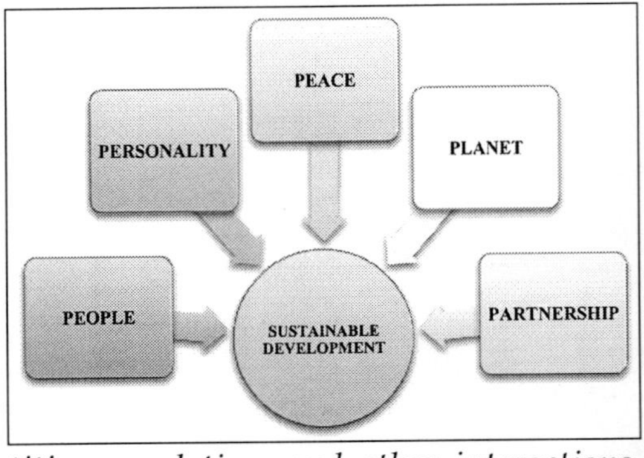


*The rapidly increasing human population and its diverse human activities have had an influence on the ecological environment, causing degradation of both*

CSIR-Indian Institute of Toxicology Research, Lucknow, Uttar Pradesh (India)
*National Green Tribunal, Lucknow, Uttar Pradesh (India)
**Department of Botany, University of Lucknow, Lucknow, Uttar Pradesh (India)
***Department of Botany, Shia Degree College, Lucknow, Uttar Pradesh (India)

*physical and biological components. Issues such as deforestation, industrialization, global warming, environmental stressors, pollution, overuse of natural resources, and pesticides have led to the destruction of the ecological environment and increased public awareness of ecology and the environment. There are several uncertainties in the relationship between the constructed ecosystem and human wellbeing. The planning, implementation and ecologically sustainable designing through new concepts of architecture may be helpful to combat environmental adversities. Integrity among urban, social, and biophysical sciences is critical for mitigating the looming challenges of climate change, green building architecture, improved design, and planning for greener cities in the twenty-first century. We need to integrate planning and environmental concerns during the implementation of developmental strategies. The* ***'polluter-pay principle'*** *of economic law may be supplemented by strict control policies as appropriate.*

*The bookchapter analyses the major environmental issues as well as the reasons for ecology's failure to provide solutions to environmental problems. It is also indicated that environmental problems are not only scientific and technological in nature but also have social and economic dimensions that must be addressed with the help of social sciences in order for human aspirations to be met in a sustainable manner.*

***Keywords:*** *Deforestation, Ecosystem, Pollution, Strategies, Sustainability, Urban.*

## INTRODUCTION

We need to undertake pledge to collectively work in harmony with nature towards conserving precious environment resources. Moreover, we respect nature as an integral part of our culture but since last few decades it is observed that the strings have loosened and needs concerted and action with true spirits. We are well aware that scientists and environmentalists may describe which factors may have an impact on the environment based on documentary evidence and data. However, the solutions are the responsibility of society as a whole.

According to Claudine Schneider, a US representative, a healthy ecology is the basis for a healthy economy. The formulation stone for a circular and strong economy must be based on sustenance with increased, techno-feasible, better lifestyle with services ranging from food and fuel, innovative packaging and clean water, pure air to breathe, and healthy soil for growing vegetation. The biological ecosystem plays a critical role in the upliftment of the economy through extrinsic and intrinsic factors, direct input into production, and many allied services. Ecological economics relates to the relationship between ecosystems and the economy. Sustainability, climate change, global warming, ozone depletion, and the extinction of biodiversity species are just a few of the issues that must be addressed.

We need a safe, healthy, and supportive eco-friendly environment for us and future generations. Our lives are dependent on the environment for energy and key natural resources for sustenance. The adequate water is vital for drinking, sanitation, and hygiene. Clean air and water, sound agricultural practices, a stable climate, and health-promoting developments in urban and rural areas could all serve as potential homes for upcoming generations. Environmental science knowledge encompasses multi-disciplinary science with more integrated approach and upgradation of transferable skills that are needed in the upcoming job market. Experienced and trained human resources are necessary to make the nature conservation process work in efficient manner.

Internationally, EPA helps regulated entities meet federal requirements, and holds entities legally accountable for violations. It also issues guidance documents to further clarify and assist in implementation of regulations. Resource Conservation and Recovery Act (RCRA) goals are to protect us from the hazards of waste disposal; conserve energy, natural resources by recycling and recovery; reduce or eliminate waste; and clean up waste that which may have spilled, leaked or been improperly disposed of indiscriminately.

During the COVID-19 pandemic, there was a major drop in greenhouse gas emissions, with a 17 percent reduction in carbon dioxide emissions by April 2020 as especially in comparison to April 2019, but the reduction in carbon dioxide emissions was temporary, and emissions climbed as soon as lockdown initiatives were lifted, as seen in China and India.

## MAJOR ECOLOGICAL ISSUES FOR THE PRESENT GENERATION WITH FAR REACHING IMPACTS

The procedural specifications or guidelines outline the core requirements and steps required for compliance with the ecological and environmental assessment process rules and regulations.

## DEFORESTATION

When trees are cut down, the carbon they are storing is released into the atmosphere, where it combines with other greenhouse gases and contributes to global warming. According to most estimates, the destruction of tropical rainforests emits more carbon dioxide into the atmosphere than all of the automobiles and trucks that travel the world's highways combined. Deforestation and degradation may be the cause of substantial carbon emissions with global impacts on the balance on the sustainability of the global climate system. The world's wide forest ecosystem is facing forest fires due to extreme drought in tropical geographical regions. Deforestation is a severe growing issue where wood is used for cooking inspite of national efforts of Ujjwala Yojna in India. In our country, nearly 38.5 thousand hectares of tropical forest declined during last few years making up nearly 5.3 to 14 per cent loss of its tree cover. The total forest cover in India (2022) is 7, 13,789 square kilometers which is 21.71% of the total geographical area.

Deforestation has reached alarming levels during last few decades and the average rate of tropical deforestation in the region was 5 million ha per year. Desertification has affected more than 860 million ha of land and 150 million people in the Asiatic region. The extraction of groundwater has caused water stressed regions throughout the globe in varied pockets with land subsidence, saltwater intrusion, and groundwater pollution.

Allen *et al.* (2010)investigated draught and head induced tree mortality in forests as a result of emerging climate change risk. In 2015, Reyer *et al,* have explained forest resilience as anthropogenic global changes with profound impacts on ecosystem function and services. Hence Deforestation not only endangers known species, but also undiscovered ones.

## INDUSTRIALIZATION

The fast-growing industrialization has created serious impacts on nature depending on the types of industrializing activity and the surrounding environment. The total vegetation cover has decreased with land usage and metal pollution has enormously increased through rapid socio-economic development. Carbon dioxide ($CO_2$) emissions are substantially lower than it was before industrialization began. Greenhouse gas (GHG) concentration levels are significantly higher than they were at the start of the industrial era, which means that atmospheric $CO_2$ concentrations reached 409.8 ppm (parts per million) in 2019, the highest level in at least 800,000 years, and is expected to reach 550 ppm in 2050.

The OECD countries and the International Energy Agency (IEA) have agreed to noticeably increase the public expenditure for energy research and development in order to reduce greenhouse gas emissions. Numerous new agreements were signed with Mission Innovation (MI) and the Clean Energy Ministry (CEM) to enhance clean energy technology and increase 100% expenditures for achievements in terms of technological areas and allied research and development. The OECD's 38 member countries have also agreed to implement the Kyoto Protocol in order to reduce greenhouse gas emissions and address global environmental issues. As a result, in order to reduce reliance on fossil fuels, OECD members have high ambitions to enhance overall R & D budgets in an attempt to optimize sources of clean energy. This is due to a 6% increase in greenhouse gas emissions from fossil fuel combustion in 2015, which is recognized as a significant reason for environmental disaster degradation in OECD countries.

Natural and human sources of $CO_2$ emissions include respiration, decomposition, cement production, transportation, natural gas extraction, fossil fuel combustion, and ocean release. The earth's average surface temperature has increased by about 0.6°C since gas emissions began, achieved its highest level in the last millennium. Carbon dioxide is a gas that lasts much longer in the atmosphere than other greenhouse gases and has been found all over the world.

## LOSS OF BIODIVERSITY

After pandemic, post covid-19 experiences globally international organizations are working to reenergize international cooperation and collective action. In the words of UN Secretary-General, "We are at a crossroads, with consequential choices before us. It can go either way: breakdown or breakthrough". According to European Commission (EC) estimates > 80 percent of the continent's habitats are in "poor" shape and repairing of ecosystems is crucial to countering climate change and saving species from extinction.

## POPULATION, POLLUTION AND POVERTY – A MENACE

The unprecedented global demographic changes have far reached economic implications due to systematic features of the human life cycle. The population's size, age structure, and geographic distribution may influence the growing economy and productivity. Per capita labor income and opportunities may differ by region. Due to economic pressures, child labor has become an integral part of society, which in turn affects the education and mental growth of the younger population. In the present scenario, India holds the second position in the population index, which is 17.7% of the total world population. Sincere efforts are vital on various sustainability measures, viz. climate change and air quality, as on the Environmental Performance Index-2022 we have a score of 18.9 and rank in the bottom 5 of the 180 countries, where Denmark is ranked first in the sustainability and environmental health categories. There are several theoretical and empirical researches on the various aspects of the poverty-environment nexus.

It is well said that poverty is a major cause and effect of global environmental problems. Several regions of the universe are caught in a vicious downwards spiral: poor people are forced to overuse environmental resources to survive from day to day, and their impoverishment of their environment further impoverishes them, making their survival difficult. As per latest approaches on the environment, aggregate environment and degradation to which 'population' and 'society' relate are challenged by ideas viz. socially-differentiated people use and value elements/aspects of environment in different ways. We need to monitor land cover change and environmental change in coastal and marine resources and potential relations with climate changes. The closed linkages between population, poverty and environment in the thickly populated regions may help to identify set of strategic directions for the future. Well known economist,Amartya Sen has been instrumental in highlighting that the issue regarding access to food, in contrast to its production, as the most important explanatory variable in food security and resilience of populations. He argues, that entitlements are actual and potential bundles of commodities which individuals can access and that most famines are cause of circumstances of entitlements, failures due to political actions. It is therefore concluded with the underlying vulnerability of societies to the poverty and resources issue in the context of population pressure.Thus, underprivileged groups instead of being agents are more often than not victims of environmental degradation and we need not fall into to trap of seeing the poor as passive. The social factors e.g., gender, poverty, inequity and conflict etc. may affect both incentives and environmental conservation.

Poverty of the population may expose women and children as most susceptible to incidence of indoor air pollution. It is felt that the increased time and energy spent in collecting biomass fuels contributes to the physical burden and ill health of women and children.

## WASTE DISPOSAL AND MANAGEMENT

For a long time, the waste that humans generate has been harmful to our environment. Humans produce far too much garbage and are incapable of dealing with it in a sustainable manner. Non-biodegradable waste that cannot be recycled properly is filling our oceans and landfills. The concept of circular economy desires the replacement of "end of life approaches with the restoration concept, use of renewable sources of energy, refusal of usage of toxicants, and reduction in waste through rearranging production and supply processes"

Globally, waste generation rates are rising and it was estimated to generate 2.24 billion tonnes of solid waste, amounting to a footprint of 0.79 kilograms per person per day in 2020. With rapid urbanization the wastegenerations per year are expected to increase by 73% and reach to 3.88 billion tonnes in 2050.

The practices of land filling or open burning, incineration etc. may create serious health, safety, and environmental impacts.Unregulated waste management practicesserve as a breeding ground for disease vectors, contributes to methane generation through climate changes. We need to managing waste and convert to wealth for building sustainable existence. The effective waste management is expensive and municipal service requires integrated systems that are efficient, sustainable, acceptable and socially supported.

## SOIL EROSION

Severe droughts triggered soil erosion and land degradation with crippling of farms and dairy animals. The fodder is insufficiently available at high prices. Erosion may be expected to continue past the construction phase on embankments and cut slopes and landslips are expected in areas of heavy rainfall. The maintenance work must include critical inspection of earthworks and drainage supply and distribution systems, and remedial actions.

### Air Pollution and EIA

The deterioration in air quality and the rapid increase of greenhouse gases are top issues of concern in view of the environment performance index. The pulmonary diseases that cause increased discomfort to people with asthma and heart diseases are directly related to the air quality index.Indeed, in many countries EIA must be an integral part of the feasibility study. Where these laws are implemented strictly, they may be a powerful means of directing development towards sustainability.This process involves site selection, screening, initial assessment, and putting terms of reference or scope as per requirements.Negative socioeconomic impacts include the appropriation of land, the weakening of existing community linkages through relocation, and the suppression of agricultural land.

Every year, adverse exposure to air pollutants leads to an estimated 7 million mature deaths. This is potentially linked to reduced lung growth, functions, and pulmonary infections and stokes in the varied age groups. Thus, burden of disease attributable to air pollution is on at par with other health risks due to unhealthy diet and smoking (active and passive). The particulate matter of 2.5 microns (μm) to 10 microns (μm) is of particular health relevance as it is capable of penetration deep into the lungs and may also enter the blood stream, leading to several health complications.

Healthy plants with extended leaves or foliage are a boon for such populations. We need to enhance forestations in different parts of the world so as to provide a cleaner and healthier environment for future generations. Some outdoor trees such as *ficus religiosa* (peepal), *azadirachta indica* (neem), *ficusbenghalensis* (banyan) and a few indoor plants like pothos plant, spider plant, areca palm, snake plant, tulsi, bamboo plant etc are good for providing oxygen.

## WATER POLLUTION: MONITORING AND MANAGEMENT

Water safety plants are being designed at the international level for risk assessment and risk management, with the goal of consistently ensuring the safety and acceptability of pure drinking water supplies across socioeconomic settings. The steps have been taken by NitiAyog to ensure and improve pipe water supplies through stake holders. The stressed condition in overpopulated areas is a critical issue from a health point of view. According to UNICEF and WHO, there are several inequalities in the accessibility of clean water, appropriate sanitation, and hygiene, with approximately one out of three people globally having no access to safe drinking water (UNICEF report 2019). In a few rural areas of India, the potable source of water ranges from 2.5 kilometers. In Rajasthan (area 3, 42,239 sq km; population 78.23 millions) more than 25% has presence of fluoride in the groundwater. This fluoride causes fluorosis, which is an irreversible disease, and the economy is primarily based on agriculture and animal husbandry.

Besides the demographic and socio-economic factors, the cast continues to play a critical role in determining access to water in a few villages, despite attempts to change behavior. Poverty aggravated water-related stress and investment in water collection and purification. The sedimentation and erosion caused by floods in some areas leads to landslides, the care of rich humus soil from agricultural lands, degradation of water quality and harmful blooms of algae, which lead to water pollution, causing harmful effects to aquatic organisms as well as plants.

The oxygen deprivation in waterlogged areas may affect the marine flora and fauna. Floods may spur on migration, dispersion, as well as become a breeding ground for mosquitoes, leading to several diseases. The large debris may cause adverse impacts through structural damage to bridges, highways, and dams. Besides, the surface and groundwater may be contaminated, making it unfit for consumption.

## CONTAMINANTS OF EMERGING CONCERN

The term "contaminants of emerging concern" (CECs) is used by experts in water quality to refer to pollutants that have been found in water bodies, may have an impact on human or ecological health, and are often not covered by present environmental legislation. Emerging contaminants (ECs) are pollutants of growing concern. The majority of them are organic substances that have recently been discovered in natural wastewater streams produced by human and industrial activities. These substances include pesticides, pharmaceuticals and personal care products, heavy metals, persistent organic pollutants, plasticizers, food additives, laundry detergents, surfactants, disinfectants, flame retardants, and other organic substances.

The European Commission initiated the NORMAN project in 2005 to promote a permanent network of reference laboratories and research centers, integrating academic institutions, industry, government regulatory bodies, and NGOs, with participation from 70 members from over 20 countries.

## PERSISTENT ORGANIC POLLUTANTS (POPs)

POPs are organic (carbon-based) compounds that do not break down easily in the environment. Persistence, long-distance migration, potential bioaccumulation, and latent toxicity are characteristics of persistent organic pollutants (POPs) that have received much attention in recent decades. There is no doubt that POPs have a negative impact on the global ecosystem. They accumulate through the food web, reaching peak concentrations of species at the top of the web, and pose a risk of harm to human health and wild animals. POP substances frequently share three characteristics, such as: one or more aromatic or aliphatic cyclical ring structures; a lack of polar functional groups; a variable amount of halogen substitutions, usually chlorine. They are typically examples of micropollutants, which are chemical compounds that can withstand degradation in the environment. The POPs include pesticides (organochlorine pesticides (OCPs), dichlorodiphenyl trichloroethanes (DDTs), aldrin, dieldrin, chlordane, endrin, heptachlor, mirex, and toxaphene), industrial chemicals (polychlorinated biphenvls (PCBs), PBDEs, hexabromocyclododecanes (HBCDs), perfluoroalkyl substances (PFASs), perfluorooctane sulphonic acid (PFOS), SCCPs, hexachlorobenzene (HCB), hexachlorocyclohexane (HCHs), aromatic hydrocarbons, and unintended by-products (dibenzodioxins and dibenzofurans).

Intentionally produced chemicals are currently or once used in agriculture, disease control, manufacturing, or industrial processes. Examples include (polychlorinated biphenyls) PCBs, which have been useful in a variety of industrial applications (e.g., in electrical transformers and large capacitors, as hydraulic and heat exchange fluids, and as additives to paints and lubricants) and dichloro-diphenyl-trichloroethane (DDT), which is still used to control mosquitoes that carry malaria in some parts of the world. Unintentionally produced chemicals, such as dioxins, that result from some industrial processes and from combustion (for example, municipal and medical waste incineration and backyard burning of trash). As a result, it is crucial to establish a simple, safe, and long-term strategy for removing POPs from water bodies. Among other conventional techniques, the adsorption process has been conclusively demonstrated to be a more effective technique for eliminating POPs and meeting discharge regulations to a greater extent.

The number of publications on adsorption applications for wastewater disposal has recently increased (from 2010 to 2021). The process has received considerable attention among the various treatment methods due to its latent efficiency, easy operation, high selectivity at the molecular level, efficiency at lower pollutant concentrations, low energy consumption, and ability to isolate multiple components. Pesticides, hydrocarbons, dyes, phenols, biphenyls, oils and greases, detergents, pharmaceuticals, and other POPs are removed from water using the adsorption mechanism.

## PHARMACEUTICALS, ANTIBIOTICSAND PERSONAL CARE PRODUCTS (PPCPs)

The presence of substances in any environmental matrix does not always imply that they are dangerous or potentially harmful. However, the discovery of substances for which there is evidence that they may negatively impact aquatic life gives rise to serious concerns. The ecosystems are experiencing increased pressure due to the emission of many classes of emerging contaminants and the interactions of these pollutants, such as bisphenols (BPs), plasticizers or pharmaceuticals are sporadic with still need to fill up the gaps in better understanding of mode of actions, quantum of pollution load, strategic planning with dynamic variability of compounds .PPCPs are found in freshwater environments at very low concentrations, but many of them, as well as their metabolites, are physiologically active and can affect aquatic organisms that are not their intended targets. The ability of PPCPs to interfere with the endocrine system may cause undesirable consequences or homeostasis disruption.

It is the need of the present times to implement state-of-the-art environmental techniques to the recognition and characterization of emerging pollutants in the aquatic environment with high sensitivity using powerful method of structural characterization, advanced mass spectrometric and chromatographic techniques. We may employ tools to meet the challenge of emerging pollutants, including pharmaceuticals and personal care products, agents of sabotage, and explosives.

The World Health Organization (WHO) defines endocrine disruptors (ED) as "exogenous substance(s) or mixture(s) that affect the function(s) of the endocrine system and thus result in detrimental health effects in an organism, its progeny, or subpopulation." EDs are a large class of chemicals found in a variety of consumer products, both natural and artificial e.g., cleaning products, antimicrobials, food preservatives, PAHs, BPA and phthalates. The possible emergence of antibiotic-resistant bacterial strains in naturally occurring bacterial populations is a significant worry associated with the availability of PPCPs in the environment. The main contributor to the emergence and spread of antibiotic resistant bacteria is the widespread use of antibiotics in human medicine and animal husbandry. This poses a threat to the efficient prevention and treatment of a number of infectious diseases brought on by antibiotic-resistant pathogenic bacteria. The predominance of R & D on DDT and its sub moieties/analogues suggests its relevance in the context of disease-vector management.

## AGROCHEMICALS

Pesticides may be categorized under different groups based on structure and specifications. They are toxic to both humans and target pests and may pass through the environment and exert adverse effects on beneficial biota and health. It may pollute the water, soil, and atmosphere of the ecosystem if estimated above than the permissible limits. The workers involved directly in production, packaging, spray or transportation may be occupationally exposed to pesticides. Pesticide exposure in the general population primarily happens through the consumption of food and water contaminated with pesticide residues; however, substantial exposure may also occur through indirect modes. Currently, intelligent, responsive, biodegradable, and biocompatible materials have attracted considerable interest through nanotechnological approaches for the formulation of green, safe, pesticides or other agrochemicals. Nano urea is receiving momentum in the present scenario due to inherent advantages. The usage of agrochemicals needs to increase food production so as to feed fast growing human population with continuous thrust on the intensive use of pesticides and fertilizers.

## HEAVY METALS

Heavy metals are naturally occurring elements with a high atomic weight and at least five times the density of water. Metals are found in abundance in nature, including rocks, ores, soil, water, and air. The unrestricted industrial use of coal, natural gas, petroleum, and waste incineration worldwide, today's humanity as well the environment is exposed to the highest level of these metals in recorded ecological history. Toxic metals are metals that form toxic soluble compounds and have no biological function; in fact, these are minerals that are toxic and have no known role in the body. They have a high density and are toxic or poisonous even in small amounts. The toxic effects of specific metals in specific forms and doses have emerged as a major cause of disease, ageing, memory loss, and even genetic defects.

The bioaccumulation of heavy metals causes a wide range of toxic impact on various body tissues and organs. Heavy metals interfere with cellular processes such as growth, proliferation, differentiation, damage repair, and apoptosis. The mechanisms of action of these metals to stimulate toxicity that are similar, including ROS generation, antioxidant defense weakness, enzyme inactivation, and oxidative stress. Some, on the other hand, have selective binding to specific macromolecules. Another significant characteristic of chronic exposure is the finding of several metals as human carcinogens. While the actual mechanism is unknown, abnormal changes in the genome and gene expression have been proposed as an underlying process. Metals that are carcinogenic, such as arsenic, cadmium, and chromium, can interfere with DNA synthesis and repair.

## ENVIRONMENTAL STRESSORS

Sustainable development is the outcome of diligently integrating environmental, economic, and social needs to attain both an improved standard of living and gain or equilibrium among human, natural, and economic resources for future generations.

Our potential of destruction may be extrapolated through the deterioration of the ozone layer, extinction of few species, and mass deforestation and desertification. In several parts of the globe, economic development projects directed at improving levels of materialistic comfort have detrimental effects on people and natural resources. The natural treasures in form of water, land, and air have degraded with direct implications on development and quality of life. The inadequate planning for environment conservation, anthropogenic activities have led to the disruption of social and communal harmony, the loss of human livelihood as well as spurring of new diseases and the destruction of renewable resources.

## ECOTOURISM AND ECO-MEDICAL OPPORTUNITIES

Countries may promote partnerships and capacity building within small businesses that rely on maintenance of biodiversity. The eco tour operators may be allowed to profit from the maintenance of natural environment and hand holding relationship with these businesses may contribute significantly to employment and investments. The protected areas are ecotourism locations of preferences and many of these areas have been created to protect biodiversity and improve human wellbeing. The growth of ecotourism activities on a global scale has led to physical damage of natural ecosystems, an increase in pollution, landscape degradation, the destruction of flora and fauna, water shortages etc.

The affordable, quality based medical procedures, services have been attracting more medical tourists to India. The medical tourism may help to tap into its ecotourism potential. Burgeoning medical tourism in different well known eco-tourism destinations help to foster the international tourism map. It is anticipated that development of healthcare infrastructure with globally-acclaimed community of medical professionals has turned India into a popular destination for medical tourism. The medical, biomedical experts, professional nursing, paramedical personnel, allied medical service sector viz nutritionists, food packaging and supply, physiotherapists, psychologists, geriatricians etc. may obtain good jobs with better salaries depending on competencies and state of art capabilities.

## JOB CAREERS FOR SKILLED ECOLOGISTS

There are several opportunities for experts or skilled manpower with specialization in ecology. It may range from field ecologist, restoration, park naturalist, marine biologists, environmental consultant, to environmental protection specialist(s) and natural resources managers. The basic and perks depends on job profile and responsibilities.The careers as environmental scientists are expected to grow 8 percent during next decade. In India, particularly in Uttarakhand, Himachal, Jammu & Kashmir, North-eastern regions and few others are regularly promoting home stays by means of a policy that provides subsidies for the initial set up and it aim to increase tourism in remote areas by increasing employment and income for home owners and curbing migration. Thus, the adventure and excitement of travel; meaningful global connections; and perhaps even a chance to explore entrepreneurial satisfaction reveals great potential.

## INFERENCE

The environmental impact assessments may play important role in resolving the environmental problems through its ability to contribute to environmentally sound and sustainable development. The restoration of degraded ecosystems is fundamental for achieving the SDGs primarily on climate change, poverty eradication, food security, water, sanitation and hygiene although all are important.Comprehensive environmental planning may help to generate sufficient data for the rational use of renewable natural resources. The sectoral development planning, national and regional conservation strategies and environmental profiles are expected to create the baseline information for environmental impact assessment. It may help in sustainable rural development based on environmental protection, creation of jobs, education and awareness about endangered animals and climate change, improvement of life quality with improved understanding, sensitivity towards other cultures etc. Our small efforts of planting trees may make the travelling environment friendly, tourist places clean and tidy. The education and awareness about endangered animals and climate change may contribute in helping the improvement of quality life and attaining sustainable development goals within the stipulated time frame.

We in coming years would need to develop micro level interventions, equitable decision-making mechanisms and participatory policy processes that ensure effective participation of the poor and marginalized groups. The laws and legislation must be stringent to address access and property rights especially around protected areas and forests so as to develop activities for poverty-environment monitoring assessment. Our government policies and subsidies' may promote high value, low impact, and other 'biodiversity-friendly' products.

Ecotourism may be well promoted as an adventure with win-win solution for resource conservation, excitements and local people dependent on those resources. The material and symbolic factors may influence farmers' decision-making regarding land use change. We need to holistically examine land use change in the context of ecotourism in rural areas given that ecotourism is presumed to have minimal impact on landscape of specific geographical regions.

## REFERENCES


1. Ahmed, F., Ali, I., Kousar, S., & Ahmed, S. (2022). The Environmental Impact of Industrialization and Foreign Direct Investment: Empirical Evidence from Asia-Pacific Region. *Environmental Science and Pollution Research, 29.* https://doi.org/10.1007/s11356-021-17560-w
2. Adger, W.N. (1999) Social Vulnerability to Climate Change and Extremes in Coastal Vietnam. World Development, 27(2), 249-269.
3. Ahmed, F., Ali, I., Kousar, S., & Ahmed, S. (2022). The Environmental Impact of Industrialization and Foreign Direct Investment: Empirical Evidence from Asia-Pacific Region. *Environmental Science and Pollution Research, 29.* https://doi.org/10.1007/s11356-021-17560-w
4. Asian Development Bank. 1993b. Environmental Assessment Requirements and Environmental Review Procedures of the Asian Development Bank. Office of the Environment, Asian Development Bank, Manila, Philippines. March 1993, 44 pp.
5. Clapp, C., Château, J., Lanzi, E., Magné, B., & Jasper Van Vliet. (2011). OECD Environmental Outlook to 2050 Climate Change Chapter pre-release version.
6. Government of the Republic of Indonesia. 1992a. Cikampek-Padalarang Toll Road Project, Environmental Impact Analysis. Ministry of Public Works, P.T. Jasa Marga (Persero), Directorate General of Highways, Indonesian Highway Corporation #Y02121-66, 133 pp.
7. Government of the Republic of Indonesia. 1992b. Cikampek-Padalarang Toll Road Project, Environmental Management Plan. Ministry of Public Works, P.T. Jasa Marga (Persero), Directorate General of Highways, Indonesian Highway Corporation #Y02121-66, 80 pp.
8. Government of the Republic of Indonesia. 1992c. Cikampek-Padalarang Toll Road Project, Environmental Monitoring Plan (RPL). Ministry of Public Works, P.T. Jasa Marga (Persero), Directorate General of Highways, Indonesian Highway Corporation #Y02121-66, 44 pp.
9. Jalal, K.F. (1993) Sustainable Development, Environment and Poverty Nexus. Occasional Papers No. 7 Asian Development Bank. Jalal, K.F. (1993) Sustainable Development, Environment and Poverty Nexus. Occasional Papers No. 7 Asian Development Bank.
10. Jalal, K.F. 1993. Sustainable Development, Environment and Poverty Nexus. Occas. Pap. No. 7. Economics and Development Resource Centre, Asian Development Bank, Manila, Philippines. December 1993. 24 pp.
11. Jodha N.S. (1992) Mountain Perspective and Sustainability: A Framework for Development Strategies. Chapter 2 in Jodha, N.S.; M. Banskota and T. Partap (eds), Sustainable Mountain Agriculture. Vol. 1 and 2, International Centre for Integrated Mountain Development. Oxford & IBH Publishing Co.
12. Jodha, N.S. (1986) "Common Property Resources and Rural Poor in Dry Regions of India", Economic and Political Weekly, 21(27): 1169-1181.
13. Jodha, N.S. (1990) "Rural Common Property Resources Contributions and Crisis." Economic and Political Weekly June 30th.
14. Jodha, N.S. (1991) "Sustainable Agriculture in Fragile Resource Zones: Technological Imperatives". Economic and Political Weekly 26: 13 A15-A26.
15. Kadekodi, G.K. ed. (1995) Operationalising Sustainable Development, Ecology Economy Interactions at a Regional Level. Internal Publication. The Netherlands: Institute for Environmental Studies (IVM).

16. Koziell, I. And Saunders, J. (2001) Living off Biodiversity: Exploring Livelihoods and Biodiversity, London: IIED.
17. Parvaneh Sobhani, Hassan Esmaeilzadeh, Seyed Mohammad Moein Sadeghi, and Marina ViorelaMarcu (2022), Estimation of Ecotourism Carrying Capacity for Sustainable Development of Protected Areas in Iran, Int J Environ Res Public Health. 2022 Feb; 19(3): 1059.
18. Sikder, M., Wang, C., Yao, X., Huai, X., Wu, L., Kwame Yeboah, F., Wood, J., Zhao, Y., & Dou, X. (2022). The Integrated Impact of GDP Growth, Industrialization, Energy use, and Urbanization on CO2 Emissions in Developing Countries: Evidence from the Panel ARDL Approach. *The Science of the Total Environment, 837,* 155795. https://doi.org/10.1016/j.scitotenv.2022.155795
19. UNDP (1998) The Human Development Report 1998, New York: UNDP. UNDP *et. al.* (2002) Linking Poverty Reduction and Environmental Management: Policy Challenges and Opportunities, Discussion Document, January 2002.
20. UNEP (1995) Poverty and the Environment: Reconciling Short Term Needs with Long Term Sustainability Goals. Kenya: UNEP.
21. World Bank (1997) Expanding the Measure of Wealth: Indicators of Sustainable Development, ESD Series No. 17, Washington D.C.: World Bank.
22. World Bank (2001) World Development Report 2000/2001 Attacking Poverty, Washington D.C.: Oxford University Press.
23. World Commission on Environment and Development (1987) Our Common Future: the Report of the World Commission on Environment and Development. Oxford: Oxford University Press. WWF Annual Report 2000.
24. WWF (2000) Trans-boundaries Collaboration at the Roof of the World. WWF, Gilgit, Pakistan: 17 pp.
25. Wikipedia Contributors. (2019, February 27). *Ecology*. Wikipedia; Wikimedia Foundation. https://en.wikipedia.org/wiki/Ecology

**Corresponding author: Prof. V.P. Sharma, CSIR-Indian Institute of Toxicology Research, Lucknow, Uttar Pradesh, India.**
**Email id: vpsitrc1@rediffmail.com**

Pages: 125-132
Emerging Environmental Contaminants and Global Healthcare Systems
*Editors:* Prof. (Dr.) Shyam Narain Pandey; Murtaza Abid
Prof. (Dr.) Syed Rais Haider; Dr. Sabiha Kazmi; Dr. Mohd. Zahid Rizvi
*ISBN:* 978-81-959169-2-4
*Edition:* 2023
*Published by:* Discovery Publishing House, New Delhi (India)

# Food Contamination
## *An Overview*

**Ananya Dhiman, Kushal Saxena, Amit Gupta**

## ABSTRACT

*Food is a pivotal part of life for healthy living and growing and for this, it is necessary to have contaminant free food to have a healthy diet. Food is a range of nutrients like water, vitamins, minerals, fats, and carbohydrates. Environmental contaminants are the substances that are toxic to living beings when they are present in high levels of the amount which may have been produced by excessive industrialisation, mining and agricultural practices. It may cause severe damage to the human body as it may experience severe headache, continuous vomiting, impaired nervous system, liver damage, heart impairment, higher or lower blood levels, lack of coordination, brain damage and paralysis. Here, we will discuss various groups which are the major contaminants of food like Polychlorinated biphenyls, Polybrominated biphenyls, mercury and methylmercury and radioactivity and the major incidents they have caused worldwide leading to a large number of patients and deaths.*

***Keywords:*** *Food; diet; contamination; patient; death.*

## INTRODUCTION

It is crucial for the living beings on this earth to survive and for this a healthy nutrition is really significant that depends on the intake of the nutritional contents. A good nutrition with physical activities is pivotal part for a healthy lifestyle which helps in decreasing the risk of diseases and

**Department of Life Sciences (Microbiology), Graphic Era Deemed to be University, Dehradun (India)**

maintaining a healthy weight. Food refers to the broad range of edible materials that comprises of essential nutrients like water, carbohydrates, fats, minerals etc., which are required for growth and living [1].

Food composition refers to the analysis of the nutrients like vitamins and minerals and substances present in the given food. Food comprises of both energy as well as non-energy components and the energy is obtained by the body in the form of calories. The chemical composition of food includes carbohydrates, fats, vitamins, proteins and minerals [2].

Water is the major component of every type of food that we eat but it also promotes bacterial growth which leads to food spoilage. the food spoilage level depends on the storage of the food which can be altered in two ways, freezing and dehydration. Vitamins are the most pivotal part of life regulating all the body functioning as nothing in the body would have exist without them. There are 13 types of vitamins: A, C, D, E, K and B (8 different type of Vitamin B). Carbohydrates are the organic compounds having carbon, hydrogen and water divided into two types: sugar and starch being the important source of energy [3]. Proteins are the basic materials in life containing hydrogen, nitrogen, oxygen and carbon as without this, no body function will perform. It can be broken down into complete or incomplete forms. Complete proteins supply 9 amino acids that are essential for the body referring to the animal proteins whereas plant proteins have all the essential amino acids [4]. Fats are insoluble in water and are composed of carbon, hydrogen and oxygen which are important for the body to function. It supplies the essential fatty acids, acids and glycerol and it also serves as a storage substance for the extra calories in body. Excess carbohydrates also turn into fats in the body [5]. Minerals are another food component important for our physique as it acts as nutrients which is helpful for the functioning of heart and digestive system. The minerals we need are boron, calcium, chloride, copper, iron, iodine, zinc, sodium, potassium etc. [1-5].

**Food contamination:** Environmental contaminants are the substances which include harmful bacterial and fungal toxins coming from the human activities like industrialisation, mining and agriculture practices such as using chemical fertilizers and pesticides. Other contaminants present in the environment includes the heavy metals, radionuclides, organic chemicals etc. Environmental food contamination results in two levels: Low-level and High-level contamination. Low-level contamination comprises of substances like polychlorinated biphenyls (PCBs). They were widely used heat-transfer fluids in transformers and capacitors and as an additive in carbon paper, dyes, pesticides and plastics but were ceased in the year 1977. High-level contamination consists of substances like polybrominated biphenyls (PBBs) that were once unintentionally mixed with the animal food and the cattle produced contaminated milk which later turned into contaminated dairy products [6].

The food gets contaminated in various ways and through distinct routes on the basis of their physical, chemical and biological properties, its usage and the source of contamination. The main way of contamination is the air-borne material on the vegetation or the soil. The organic substances are either from the industries or agriculture practices where the pesticides are the only one known as agriculture chemicals and are environmental contaminants of the food. Although, the pesticides can only contaminate the food when its present in it. If not properly cleaned and disinfected then the other sources of food can be the infected railways, cars, trucks, ships, storage buildings where the food is stored for a long time [7, 8]. Nuclear reactors usually do not contaminate but if accidently released, they can infect the vegetation by seeping in the ground or through leaves and water and hence lead to the high-level contamination. Gas release contains the volatile elements iodine and tritium or volatile precursors Strontium-90 and cesium-137. Metals and metallic salts can be spread through mining and refining activities. Trace metals like Cadmium present in the sewage sludge used as a fertilizer in agricultural land are the major concern for the contamination. The radionuclide is either absorbed or metabolized the biotic components of the environment. Radium dissolves with the ground water and contaminates the soil as well the vegetation [7, 8].

## HUMAN ILLNESS DUE TO CONTAMINATED FOOD

The consumption of contaminated food poses a great risk and it is a challenging to evaluate the environmental contaminants in the food. The toxicity of the substance in food, the level of substance added in food, the susceptibility of the population and the quantity in which the food is present affects the measurable health. In Japan, contamination of food with polychlorinated biphenyls (PCBs), mercury, cadmium have resulted in human illness and death. United States have been exposed to variety of contaminants through food, water and air but at low levels of PCBs, mercury and ionizing radiations [9, 10]. The following sectors summarize the current knowledge and ambiguity on health effects of these environmental contaminants.

**Polychlorinated Biphenyls:** Polychlorinated biphenyls are the class of man-made chlorinated organic chemicals used in the industries. They were mainly used in the commercial industries including electrical and heat-transfer equipment. Accumulation in the food chain, direct interaction with food and animal feeds or contact with food packing materials made up of recycled paper comprising PCBs results in environmental contamination of polychlorinated biphenyls in the food. Presently, there is a ban of PCBs due to the scientific evidence that they adversely pollute the environment as well becomes the major reason of food contamination. They do not degrade in the environment as they are lipophilic, instead they enter the adipose tissues of the humans. PCBs cause the human infection at much complex levels than those occurred in The United States. They suffered the unintended infection of edible rice-bran oil in the early part of year 1968 which led to the prevalent poisoning in the Japanese families who consumed the oil. This disease was named Yusho or the rice-oiled disease. It comes up with indications of having chloracne, eye discharge, skin discolouration, headache, fatigue, abdominal pain, menstrual changes and may lead to liver damage. The babies who were born to mothers suffering from this disease were abnormally small and had skin discolouration problems [11, 12].

On June 7, 1968 the first symptom of Yusho disease was discovered and later on 1,291 cases were reported till May 1975. Although, the polychlorinated dibenzofuran (PCDF) is present in rice oil making it contaminated, it is difficult to discuss the exact exposure to humans from the Yusho data. Some surveys convey that the PCDF makes the rice oil twice or thrice times more toxic than it is expected from the PCB content alone. In May 1975, cancer disease was attributed and it was concluded that the cancer cannot be inferred because of the high-level concentration of PCDF in the oil. There were two important results according to The Yusho study: First, the PCBs can be transmitted from the mother to the foetus and through breast feeding. Second, the PCB compounds that are highly chlorinated are excreted from the body more slowly than the less chlorinated ones. Cancer have been produced in mice and rats that were fed food with PCBs whereas monkeys who ate the contaminated food developed same reproductive disorders. Young monkeys who were breastfed by their mothers were observed to have toxic effects and abnormal behaviour [11, 12].

**Polybrominated Biphenyls:** Polybrominated Biphenyls are the man-made class of chemicals used in producing the electronic devices. They are stable substances, resistant to heat, acids, bases and oxidation and are also known as fire retardants. Exposure to high levels, PBBs cause hypothyroidism, endocrine system damage, damaged immune system and abnormalities. According to the studies, every Michigan resident have been exposed to the Polybrominated Biphenyls containing food products. The heaviest exposure received was to the 2,000 families who consumed the contaminated products from their own farm. Fries studied that if the contaminated milk intake is considered alone, then the Michigan residents were most strictly exposed to 5-15 grams over 230 days. The ones who unintentionally consumed contaminated meat or eggs, were highly affected by PBB but there were a smaller number of cases regarding this. The lower peninsula was having the most exposure than any other place. Michigan Department of Public Health in the year 1976 studied PBB absorptions in breast milk and the results came to be as expected. 96% of 53 women selected from Lower Peninsula and 43% of 42 women from the Upper Peninsula excreted PBB in their breast milk [11-13].

Wolff et al reported that the PBB was higher in males than in females as males may consume more contaminated food and have more direct connection with PBB in comparison to females and was observed was done that the young males had greater concentrations than the older females. The individual after eating PBB contaminated food experienced the symptoms like fatigue, hypersomnia, decrease in capacity in physical and mental work, headache, irritation, swelling and pain in the joints, pain in movement, severe gastrointestinal and skin problems [13].

**Mercury and Methylmercury:** The heavy metals include metalloids that have high atomic weight and density that exist in the environment. Heavy metals are classified into types: Essential and Non-essential metals. Essential metals are present in small quantities in our bodies that look after the functioning of the body. Non-essential metals like mercury are toxic and negatively affects the human body. The occurrence of the mercury or methylmercury can be both natural or anthropogenic substances which can be caused by natural activities like earthquakes, volcanic eruptions, or natural seeps. Major source of human exposure to mercury is food and it depends upon the food type, the mercury concentration in the air in that area and the use of mercury in the agricultural and industrial production of food. The living organisms and the vegetable tissues have the at least some trace amounts as they have the capability to concentrate mercury. The effects of mercury and methylmercury becomes detectable at 20 to 50μg/100ml blood level, 50 to 120mg/ kg at hair levels and 0.5 to 0.8mg/ kg body burdens between body weight [15, 16].

The widely stated exposure risk is the brain damage to the humans. Mercury gathers in the Central Nervous System and the reduction of mercury amounts in blood gets slow resulting in organizational changes of the nervous system. The indications include headache, vertigo, ataxia, pain, numbness and vasomotor disturbances which were detected in the Minamata Bay and Niigata tragedy in Japan. The first case described about congenital Minamata disease was in 1950s which observed the placental transfer of mercury and methylmercury. The transmission of mercury levels from pregnant women to the placenta is significant but if the levels are not toxic during the pregnancy, it may still give rise to the offspring with birth defects. It results in high blood levels in the babies more than it is in the mothers. In 1959, the infants born with these defects were behaving abnormally, had motor disorders which concluded that they were suffering from the cerebral palsy or cerebral dysfunction syndrome. The symptoms included lack in coordination, speaking and hearing; chewing and swallowing impairment, involuntary actions and forced laughing [15, 16].

**Radioactivity:** Radioactivity is the emission of particles occurring spontaneously where a small amount of radiation seems to be harmless. When radioactive elements decay, it causes the emission of ionizing radiation which further leads to the liver tissues damage. Heavy exposure to the ionizing radiation like X-rays, gamma rays and beta rays produce birth defects, mutations and cancers to humans which are related to the high blood levels. Less than one ionization is produced in one cell nucleus per day by the radiation levels and as cells have the capacity to repair the ionization damage, it may take low radiation exposure to restore it. Some examples of radioactive elements are:

- **Strontium-90:** It has a similar action like calcium in the body and has a long half-life. If the calcium in the body is replaced with the Strontium-90, the tissues the cells covering the bones are exposed to the radiation.
- **Iodine:** Iodine is a dangerous and short-lived emission product having a half-life of 8.02 days. The radioiodine produced in the atmosphere by nuclear power stations is taken up and concentrated by thyroid gland increasing the risk of thyroid cancer.
- **Tritium:** Tritium also called radioactive hydrogen combines chemically with oxygen to form water.

## FOOD CONTAMINATION INCIDENTS

The food contamination which includes addition of hazardous substances in the food have deadly consequences. Here are some food contamination incidents [17, 18]

1. **Morigana Dried Milk Poisoning:** This incident happened with the Morigana milk Company in Tokushima, Japan in the year 1956 where arsenic was accidently added to disodium phosphate and was later added to the milk powder. People suffered from diarrhoea, vomiting. It caused at least 100 deaths and 13,400 people affected.
2. **Minamata Bay Tragedy:** Minamata disease affects the nervous system which is caused by the mercury poisoning. Patients experience symptoms like uncontrolled actions, weakened muscles, impaired senses which further led to paralysis, madness, coma and death. It was first seen during the 1950s in one of the coastal cities in Japan when people ate contaminated sea creatures which were consumed by the humans or animals. According to the data, there were more than 2,000 people who suffered from the diseases and nearly 1,700 people died out of them.
3. **Poison Grain Disaster:** In Iraq, ingestion of toxic grain infected with mercury-based fungicide in the year 1971 resulted in 6,500 total cases reported regarding this. These grains were imported from U.S. and Mexico which was meant to be grown, not eaten. But, due to the difficulty in understanding the foreign-language labels, the rural Iraqis ate it. This disturbing incident resulted in loss of coordination, decreased sensation in the skin, eyesight loss and even brain damage.
4. **Milk Scandel:** In the Chinese Gansu Province, this deadly outbreak was out in the year 2008. Due to this, 16 babies were first testified with the kidney stone problem after consuming the powdered milk

factory-made by the dairy company Sanlu Group. When investigated, it was found that the melamine was mixed with the milk powder to make it appear higher in protein. By the end of year 2008, there were total 3,00,000 individuals, out of which 54,000 babies were admitted to the hospital. The government officials later took action in executing the case.

## ECONOMIC IMPACT

The economic impact includes the cost of the food and the health costs. The level of economic impact depends upon the amount of food contaminated, the concentration of the food contaminant, the chemical and toxic characteristics of the infectant and the action taken of the contamination of food. A single food-borne disease can affect the whole food or beverage industry by gradually decreasing their sales or even making the products eliminate from the market. The Federal and State authorities take up the primary action which can be the issuing of a cautioning of an action level or the tolerance. This establishes a permitted level for the food contaminant and if any food is found to be concentrated above the limited level, it is either demolished or constrained from being in the market. The action level or the tolerance is important because if no action level will be present then no food would be condemned and this depends upon the concentration of substances present in the food. Here, the chemical properties are equally important as its presence in the environment above the limited level will contaminate food to a great level increasing dangerous risks of diseases.

## CONCLUSION

Excess industrialisation in the world has resulted in the entry of toxic materials in the surrounding which has drastically increased risks of diseases all over the world. Food contamination has been a worldwide problem since ages with an unknown level. Even low exposure to the contaminants for a longer time gives increases the toxicity in the body. Monitoring the food contaminants as well as decreasing or eliminating the contaminants release in the environment is necessary. The general awareness about the healthy diet, proper hygiene near food, proper agricultural practices, livestock rearing and appropriate cooking methods is very important. Implementing more food safety laws is now obligatory for decreasing more and more dangerous contaminants from the environment and has a healthy lifestyle among the population.

## REFERENCES

1. Jung S, Rickert D, Deak N, Aldin E, Recknor J, Johnson L, Murphy P. Comparison of Kjeldahl and Dumas methods for Determining Protein Contents of Soybean Products. J Am Oil Chem Soc 2003; 80: 1169.

2. Norhayati MK, Mohd F, Mohd N, Nazline MK, Aswir AR, Wan S, Norliza AH, Janarthini S, Rusidah S. Individual and Total Sugar Contents of 83 Malaysian Foods. J Food Res 2018; 7: 58-63.
3. Elmadfa I, Meyer AL. Importance of Food Composition Data to Nutrition and Public Health. Eur J Clin Nutr 2010; 64 (Suppl. S3): S4-S7.
4. Zhang F, Tapera TM, Gou J. Application of a New Dietary Pattern Analysis method in Nutritional Epidemiology. BMC Med Res Methodol 2018; 18:119.
5. Montesano D, Cossignani L, Giua L, Urbani E, Simonetti MS, Blasi F. A Simple HPLC-ELSD method for Sugar Analysis in Goji Berry. J Chem 2016; 2016: 6271808.
6. Bae YJ, Kim SK. Low Dietary Calcium is associated with Self-rated Depression in Middle-aged Korean Women. Nutr Res Pract 2012; 6 (6): 527-533.
7. Ali H, Khan E, Ilahi I. Environmental Chemistry and Ecotoxicology of Hazardous Heavy Metals: Environmental Persistence, Toxicity, and Bioaccumulation. J Chem 2019; 1-14.
8. Almeida S, Raposo A, Almeida-González M, Carrascosa C. Bisphenol A: Food Exposure and Impact on Human Health Compr Rev Food Sci Food Saf 2018; 17: 1503-1517.
9. Azad MAK, Sarker M, Li T, Yin J. Probiotic species in the modulation of Gut Microbiota: An Overview. Biomed Res Bar Int 2018; 1-8.
10. Barzegar F, Kamankesh M, Mohammadi A. Heterocyclic Aromatic Amines in Cooked Food: A Review on Formation, Health Risk-toxicology and their Analytical Techniques. Food Chem 2019; 280: 240-254.
11. Aken BV, Correa PA, Schnoor JL. Phytoremediation of Polychlorinated Biphenyls: New Trends and Promises. Environ Sci Technol 2009; 44: 2767-2776.
12. Alder AC, Haggblom MM, Oppenheimer SR, Young L. Reductive Dechlorination of Polychlorinated Biphenyls in Anaerobic Sediments. Environ Sci Technol 1993; 27: 530-538.
13. Zhuang Y, Ahn S, Seyfferth AL, Masue-Slowey Y, Fendorf S, Luthy RG. Dehalogenation of Polybrominated diphenyl ethers and polychlorinated biphenyl by bimetallic, impregnated, and nanoscale zerovalent iron. Environ Sci Technol 2011; 45: 4896-4903.
14. Eriksson P, Jakobsson E, Fredriksson A. Developmental Neurotoxicity of Brominated Flame-retardants, Polybrominated diphenyl ethers and tetrabromo-bis-phenol A. Organohalogen Compds 1998; 35: 375-377.
15. Akerblom S, Bishop K, Bjorn E, Lambertsson L, Eriksson T, Nilsson MB. Significant interaction effects from Sulfate Deposition and Climate on Sulfur Concentrations Constitute major Controls on Methylmercury Production in Peatlands. Geochimica et Cosmochimica Acta 2013; 102: 1-11.
16. Bailey LT, Mitchell CPJ, Engstrom DR, Berndt ME, Coleman Wasik JK, Johnson NW. Influence of Pore Water Sulfide on Methylmercury Production and Partitioning in Sulfate-impacted Lake Sediments. Science of the Total Environment 2017; 580: 1197-1204.
17. Kantiani L, Llorca M, Sanchís J, Fare M. Emerging Food Contaminants: A Review. Anal Bioanal Chem 2010; 398: 2413-2427.
18. Liang B, Scammon D. Food Contamination incidents: What do Consumers Seek Online? Who cares? Int J Nonprofit Volunt Sect Market 2016; 21: 227-241.

**Corresponding author: Dr Amit Gupta, Associate Professor, Department of Biotechnology, Graphic Era (Deemed to be) University, Dehradun, India.**
**Email id: dr.amitgupta.bt@geu.ac.in**

Pages: 133-140
**Emerging Environmental Contaminants and Global Healthcare Systems**
*Editors:* **Prof. (Dr.) Shyam Narain Pandey; Murtaza Abid**
**Prof. (Dr.) Syed Rais Haider; Dr. Sabiha Kazmi; Dr. Mohd. Zahid Rizvi**
*ISBN:* **978-81-959169-2-4**
*Edition:* **2023**
*Published by:* **Discovery Publishing House, New Delhi (India)**

# Environmental Contaminants
## *Review*

**Kushal Saxena, Ananya Dhiman, Amit Gupta**

### ABSTRACT

*The constituents which are present in the environment above the limited concentration altering the surroundings by its toxicity affecting humans, animals, and plants are known as the environmental constituents. They are any physical, chemical, biological or radiological agents that has affects the air, water, soil, and living beings. Various types of contaminants have polluted our environment due to the overuse of chemical fertilizers and industrialization. These contaminants consist of solid, liquid, and gas particles which are produced by human activities for their economic advantages. The sources of contaminants can be classified into two types: point sources and non-point sources. A wide range of chemicals contaminates the land, water and air from industries, chemical or oil spills, from roads, wastewater treatment plants, and sewage treatment plants. The contaminants may be natural or man-made (xenobiotic) in nature. Industries, heavy metals, fossil fuels, organic agents, inorganic solvents, oil spills, mining, polyaromatic hydrocarbons, and war agents are the common sources of environmental contaminants.*

***Keywords:*** *Environment; contaminants; sources; hydrocarbons; industries.*

## INTRODUCTION

An environment is everything that surrounds us referring to all the living and non-living beings present such as soil, water, etc. The environment comes from the French word "environ" meaning surrounding. The

---

**Department of Life Sciences, Graphic Era Deemed to be University, Dehradun (India)**

environment covers the biotic and abiotic components in the surrounding where biotic components include all the living beings that are flora and fauna while the abiotic components comprise all non-living things in the surrounding like the sun, water, soil, and temperature. It endures life by providing genetics and biodiversity as it enhances the quality of living where there is no human activity in the surroundings [1, 2]. The environment helps in getting purged from the garbage that is activated by the production and consumption of resources by various industries. Environmental resources play an important role in human physical and mental well-being possessing both instrumental and fundamental characteristics. The components of the environment include the atmosphere, hydrosphere, lithosphere and biosphere which make up the majority of the environment. When it comes to the environment, we are referring to the ecosystem that is making up the atmosphere. An ecosystem is a community where biotic and abiotic elements interact with each other but the environment is different from the ecosystem as it includes the biological community where the biotic and abiotic components interact with each other. The ecosystem and the environment are like the two sides of the same coin despite being different from each other [3, 4].

The environment can be divided into the natural or geographical environment which includes land, mountains, valleys, oceans, volcanoes, deserts, forests, the natural environmental conditions like sunlight, temperature, humidity, rainfall, flora and fauna, etc. Man-made or social environment refers to the modifications in the environment like houses, cities etc. the man-made environment can be further divided into two types: Inner environment refers to the environment that undergoes as long as social values [1-5]. It is an important factor for living beings to exist. The outer environment is the surrounding that is produced by man through science and technology. It includes houses, buildings, infrastructures, transport and communication and so it can be termed as an evolving environment as it is man-made and continuous modifications are made by them. Some depleted resources are unreasonably utilized by humans leading to their extinction. Based on this, natural resources are divided into renewable and non-renewable resources. Human being uses these resources for their convenience which damages natural resources and the earth is not able to revive such kinds of resources. These kinds of resources are called non-renewable resources such as fossil fuels, natural ores and nuclear propellants like natural gas. On the other hand, renewable resources have an insignificant impact on the environment. These emissions emit low carbons upon their usage. These are resources that can revive themselves. That is why they do not get diminished. The environment provides resources for production as it contains renewable and non-renewable resources such as soil, sun, etc [2-7].

## CONTAMINANTS

The types of pollutants or contaminants found in the environment [8, 9] are as follows.

**Air Pollutants:** Air pollution can be the impact of indoor or outdoor activities by any physical, chemical, or biological agent that changes the natural environment. The air contaminants may be in solid or liquid state in the form of dust particles, smoke, oil mist etc. are visible to us. There are two types of air pollutants: Primary pollutants that directly cause the air pollution directly such as gases emitted from the industries and a Secondary pollutant that interact and reacts with the primary pollutants. Household devices, motorcycles, industrial services, forest fires etc. are common sources of air pollution. The contaminants that give a risk to the health includes particulate matter, ozone, carbon monoxide, ammonia, sulphur dioxide, nitrogen dioxide and radioactive pollutants and are highly toxic pollutants released in the air. Another source may be greenhouse gases emissions which are considered to be the major drivers of air contaminants. The effect of these emissions leads to an increase in sea levels, temperature rise, and unpredictable weather. Humans get affected a great extent by air pollution as it causes cardiovascular diseases, lung diseases, cancer, and changes the central nervous system [8, 9].

**Water Pollutants:** Water pollution is caused due to the presence of harmful substances in the water and it's no longer available for different purposes. The polluted water is toxic for both environment and the living beings. Water pollutants are the substances that can change the characteristics of water in any physical, chemical and biological forms negatively affecting the quality of water. Domestic wastes, industrial releases, agricultural waste, dumping of wastes, atmosphere (acid rain), mines, sewage waste are the common sources of the water pollution. Industrial process is one of the major sources of the water pollution. Likewise, if the polluted water is seeped into the ground, it can affect the ground water so it gets polluted in distinct ways. The sources of water pollution are divided into two: Point sources which include waste-water effluent and sewage discharge affecting the area near it and non-point sources spread over large areas by initiating from diverse places. The gastrointestinal diseases, reproductive issues, neurological disorders and even cancer are caused by the water pollution. These include Cholera, Amoebiasis, Dysentery, Diarrhoea, Hepatitis A, Lead poisoning, Polio, Malaria, Polyomavirus infections, Intestinal worms, Arsenicosis, Fluorosis, Guinea worm diseases, Trichoma, Typhoid and Schistosomiasis [8, 9].

**Soil Pollutants:** Soil pollution refers to the contamination of soil with toxic substances above the limited level. Soil pollutants can easily penetrate into the soil. The soil pollution can be caused by agricultural chemicals such as pesticides or herbicides, accidental oil spills, decreased soil fertility, acid rain, excessive industrial activity or due to the poor management of discarding the waste in soil. Fossil fuels may lead to the cause of soil pollution involving the refineries, petrochemical plants and motor vehicles. The transportation of soil pollutants can occur between the biotic and abiotic components in the environment where abiotic components show the strongest effects in transporting the soil pollutants. Air is one of the effective ways in which the soil pollutants are dispersed but it only transfers the small particles and the bigger particles are carried by the strong winds. Water is counted as another route whereas other routes include erosion and mass wasting like earthquakes, slope steepness and decreased vegetation. Using excess of pesticides or herbicides makes soil lose its fertility and change its acidity or alkalinity, hence, degrading the original quality of soil. Skin problems or respiratory diseases are caused due to working, living and playing in the soil which leads to irritation in eyes and nose, headaches, nausea, vomiting, continuous coughing and chest pain. Long term diseases include cancer, kidney and liver damage, central nervous system damage [8, 9].

## HUMAN EXPOSURE TO ENVIRONMENTAL CONTAMINANTS

The aspects of human exposure are important for studying the health-related consequences [10, 11]. These include magnitude, duration and frequency. Magnitude is an important aspect as it is said to be directly proportional to the health outcome and the frequency of exposure can have serious implications. It is essential to further know about the duration of the exposure. The specific concentration for 5 minutes is likely to be different from the same concentration for an hour.

## IMPORTANCE OF MONITORING HUMAN EXPOSURE

Exposure assessment is important to identify, evaluate and control risks in the environment. The increase in the detection of human exposure to the environment has helped in detection of hazardous agents which causes serious diseases. Human exposure trends are important because of few reasons [10-13]:

1. To understand the human population being visible to the contaminants in the environments helping identify the contaminants of possible public health awareness and the population of any group of age, race etc, who may be exposed indirectly to the contaminants of the environment
2. Tracking environmental contaminants levels in a population allowing the estimation of different ways in which the contaminants are changing in the population over time.

## MEASURES OF HUMAN EXPOSURE

Human gets in contact with many pollutants on day-to-day basis. Some of the pollutants are harmless and some are very toxic. The assessment of these contaminants is really important to study the adverse effects in the environment and to decrease the risk of harmful diseases. The measurement of human contact with the environment includes the techniques that provide quantitative and qualitative data. The exposure of human to the contaminants can be measured in a particular environment (air, water, land), with the idea of human interaction, or after the entry of contaminants in the human body through eyes, nose, skin etc. There are many ways in which the estimation of the level of human exposure is taken with both benefits and the drawbacks [11-15]. They include ambient concentration measurements, exposure modelling, personal monitoring, and biomonitoring.

1. **Ambient concentrations:** The ambient concentration measures give the information about the contaminants in the environment coming in contact with humans. In some cases, the concentration can be estimated rather than being measured. This kind of exposure estimated has given a valued substance for many regulatory and non- regulatory actions. These measurements are presented in the air, water and land but they cannot be directly connected to the monitoring indicators.
2. **Exposure modelling:** The information regarding the environmental contaminants' concentration is combined to estimate the exposure models with the help of people's activities and locations to calculate the contact of contaminants. Data is required in approach on different contaminant levels where people, live, work, play as well as get knowledge about their day-to-day activities. For the comparative toxicity of environmental contaminants, the exposures can be modelled within the chemical groups. The development of exposure indices is done to estimate the relative changes in environmental contaminant exposure over time.
3. **Personal monitoring:** With personal monitoring device, only a small number of peoples' exposure can be measured. A person wears a monitoring device during the normal days as it provides the valuable insights into the contaminants' source to which people are exposed to. They are commonly used in workplaces. The extent of sampling is enough to represent the population that is being studied and is considered as a challenge.
4. **Biomonitoring:** Biomonitoring measures the "biomarkers" referred to the contaminants, metabolites or the reaction product(s) present in the human body. Measurements are usually made up in urine or blood, but can also be taken in other various ways, such as faeces, breastmilk, hair, nails, air exhaled, as well as tissues gained from the biopsy or the autopsy. Various environmental contaminants which include heavy

metals, pesticides, and several organic pollutants can gather up in the body. This technique has been used to illustrate the exposure for many years. Recently, biomonitoring has allowed the measurement of many other environmental contaminants.

## ROE INDICATORS

ROE indicators are the simple measures that track the state of environment and human health. It represents one exposure modelling indicator and seven biomonitoring indicators. These indicators show the current status and historical trends in land, air, water, human exposure and health and the ecological condition globally [16].

## EXPOSURE MONITORING INDICATOR

To sustenance the dietary risk assessment, EPA models pesticide exposure to food using examined data sources, tools, and methods. Using this same approach, EPA changes exposure indices, which allows comparison of relative exposure to selected pesticide groups in food to a base year? This consolidative approach considers various factors that influence the exposure to pesticide, including toxicity, measured pesticide remainder levels, and food consumption information. The exposures to pesticide residues that are toxic reflect the indices and are more frequently detected at higher temperatures or are highly consumed foods. Each year, the index values are connected to the base year and indirectly evaluate the exposure, risk or cumulative risk. Measuring the relative change in pesticide exposure over a period of time is offered by these index values.

### Biomonitoring Indicators [12-16]

The biomonitoring indicators offer a total representation of selected contaminant, metabolites, human fluid levels. On a national scale, these indicators improve understanding of the extent to which exposure to individual constituents has occurred. The computable levels of various types of contaminants appear in at least some subgroup of the populations tested.

Even though ROE biomonitoring indicators reveal the comparative amounts of environmental contaminants in people and in subpopulations over a period of time, by themselves, biomarkers of exposure do not:

- Reveal information about the source of the contaminants.
- Predict whether the presence of the contaminant in the body will result in biological alterations or injurious health effects, either it is alone or acting with other contaminants in combination.
- Provide information about when, where, and how the exposure has occurred. For example, lead in children's blood may come from exposure to airborne sources, contaminated water or food, or contaminated soil or dust, but there can be no particular answer for that.
- Explain possible differences among some subpopulations.

Similarly, there are still some impurities for which there is no biomonitoring indicator and some other are not possible to analyse in the current technology of these biomonitoring indicators. These can include radon, ozone, nitrogen oxide, carbon dioxide, etc. that are some air pollutants and biological agents like molds, bacteria, viruses, dust particles. In certain cases, in certain cases, these contaminants can be bio-monitored and results will either be cost-prohibitive or not yet feasible for technology.

The evolution of biomonitoring method made the addition of exposure indicators over the time as data became available. The National Health and Nutrition Examination Survey (NHANES), for example, as a part of this, CDC adds environmental contaminants to its biomonitoring efforts. Moreover, EPA in advance will be adding various contaminants to the ROE biomonitoring indicator in upcoming future years.

## REFERENCES

1. Abnet C. Carcinogenic Food Contaminants. Cancer Invest 2007; 25: 189-196.
2. Baeumner A. Biosensors for Environmental Pollutants and Food Contaminants. Anal Bioanal Chem 2003; 377: 434-445.
3. Moores FC. Climate Change and Air Pollution: Exploring the Synergies and Potential for Mitigation in Industrializing Countries. Sustainability 2009; 1: 43-54.
4. Eze IC, Schaffner E, Fischer E, Schikowski T, Adam M, Imboden M, *et al*. Long-term Air Pollution exposure and Diabetes in a Population-based Swiss cohort. Environ Int 2014; 70: 95-105.
5. Manucci PM, Franchini M. Health Effects of Ambient Air Pollution in Developing Countries. Int J Environ Res Public Health 2017; 14: 1048.
6. Guo Y, Zeng H, Zheng R, Li S, Pereira G, Liu Q, *et al*. The Burden of Lung Cancer Mortality Attributable to Fine Particles in China. Total Environ Sci 2017; 579: 1460-6.
7. Kan H, Chen R, Tong S. Ambient Air Pollution, Climate Change, and Population Health in China. Environ Int 2012; 42: 10-9.
8. Parajuli I, Lee H, Shrestha KR. Indoor Air Quality and Ventilation Assessment of Rural Mountainous Households of Nepal. Int J Sust Built Env 2016; 5: 301-11.
9. Dockery DW, Pope CA, Xu X, Spengler JD, Ware JH, Fay ME, *et al*. An Association between Air Pollution and Mortality in Six U.S. cities. N Engl J Med 1993; 329: 1753-9.
10. Stansfeld SA. Noise Effects on Health in the Context of Air Pollution Exposure. Int J Environ Res Public Health 2015; 12: 12735-60.
11. D'Amato G, Pawankar R, Vitale C, Maurizia L. Climate Change and Air Pollution: Effects on Respiratory Allergy. Allergy Asthma Immunol Res 2016; 8: 391-5.
12. Watson JT, Gayer M, Connolly MA. Epidemics after Natural Disasters. Emerg Infect Dis 2007; 13: 1-5.
13. Wilson WE, Suh HH. Fine Particles and Coarse Particles: Concentration Relationships Relevant to Epidemiologic Studies. J Air Waste Manag Assoc 1997; 47: 1238-49.
14. Heal MR, Kumar P, Harrison RM. Particles, Air Quality, Policy and Health. Chem Soc Rev 2012; 41: 6606-30.

15. Soon W, Baliunas SL, Robinson AB, Robinson ZW. Environmental Effects of Increased Atmospheric Carbon dioxide. Climate Res 1999; 13: 149-64.
16. Abdel-Shafy HI, Mansour MSM. A Review on Polycyclic Aromatic Hydrocarbons: Source, Environmental Impact, Effect on Human Health and Remediation. Egypt J Pet 2016; 25: 107-23.

**Corresponding author: Dr. Amit Gupta, Associate Professor, Department of Biotechnology, Graphic Era (Deemed to be) University, Dehradun, India.**
**Email id: dr.amitgupta.bt@geu.ac.in**

Pages: 141-161
**Emerging Environmental Contaminants and Global Healthcare Systems**
*Editors:* **Prof. (Dr.) Shyam Narain Pandey; Murtaza Abid**
**Prof. (Dr.) Syed Rais Haider; Dr. Sabiha Kazmi; Dr. Mohd. Zahid Rizvi**
*ISBN:* **978-81-959169-2-4**
*Edition:* **2023**
*Published by:* **Discovery Publishing House, New Delhi (India)**

# Bioremediation as an Expedient Biotechnological Strategy for the Mitigation of Phenolics

**Murtaza Abid and S.N. Pandey**

**ABSTRACT**

*Bioremediation is an attractive biotechnological tool for the treatment of water and effluents containing toxic pollutants, including phenolics, which are very hazardous pollutants due to their high toxicity and environmental persistence. Several bacterial strains are used for biodegradation or biotransformation of these compounds, as an ecofriendly technology to treat contaminated environments. Most of these bacteria can utilize phenolics as sole carbon and energy source and the metabolic pathways implicated in this process are well established. Immobilization of bacterial cells on different support matrices represents a very important advance in the application of bioremediation. Furthermore, the use of this strategy and the design of new types of bioreactors would allow remediating great volumes of highly contaminated water and effluents. Due to the continuous release of industrial wastewater the application and improvement of different strategies could be very useful. This PROJECT REPORT highlights the more recent applications of bacteria for phenol bioremediation, new advances for the improvement of this technology as well as the less explored aspects that must be deepened to assess the feasibility of phenolics bioremediation from highly contaminated water and effluents.*

***Keywords:*** *Bioremediation, Biotechnological strategy, Contaminated water, Toxic pollutants, and Bacterial cells.*

**Department of Botany, University of Lucknow, Lucknow, (U.P.,) India**

## INTRODUCTION

Phenol and its derivatives represent a large group of chemical compounds consisting of a hydroxyl functional group (–OH) attached to an aromatic hydrocarbon group, with a ring structure like that of benzene. They are considered as priority pollutants because of their adverse effects on animal and human health, widespread diffusion and persistence in the environment. Their origin may be natural or anthropogenic. Phenols may occur naturally in water and soil as degradation products of lignin, one of the main components of plant cell walls. However, human activities are responsible for the main introduction of phenolics into the environment. In fact, phenolic compounds have broad spectrum of domestic, agricultural and industrial usage and they are widely used as the components of dyes, polymers, drugs and other organic substances. Industrial phenol production is estimated to be over three million tons per year, being used mostly in petrochemical industry, synthesis of resins, pharmaceuticals, perfumes, as well as intermediates in the preparation of other chemicals (e.g., plastics, drugs, explosives, pesticides and detergents), solvents or lubricating oils. Due to their high production and usage, phenolics arise as wastes or byproducts of the above mentioned industries and are widely found in the environment. In this sense, phenol is considered as an important degradation product of substituted phenols.

Moreover, chlorophenols may be formed as by-products during the disinfection of water by chlorination and as a result of the natural chlorination of organic material. Phenols are also released through automobile exhaust, fireplaces, cigarette smoke, and gases from incinerators. Although they are not release directly into water, their transference to aquatic systems may occur and high levels of these compounds have been found in the rain and, also, in fog and cloud. Measured values of phenolics in the environment show a wide range of variability depending on the precedence. For instance, phenol concentrations from petroleum refinery effluents vary between 50 and 2000 mg $L^{-1}$ for distillation units while in waste solutions generated from coal conversion processes phenols concentrations of 200-600 mg $L^{-1}$ are usually detected. Moreover, it can be assumed that phenols levels will increase over time if more stringent regulations are not taken to prevent its discharge. Phenol is included in the class 2 water hazardous pollutants list in several countries. A phenol concentration of 1 mg $L^{-1}$ or greater, affects aquatic life and may represent a risk to human health. Therefore, in most cases the accepted limit for effluents is less than 0.5 mg $L^{-1}$. In this sense, the US-EPA and WHO have established a limit concentration of 1 μg $L^{-1}$ while the European Community defined a limit of 5 μg $L^{-1}$ for phenolic compounds in drinking water. However, phenols are frequently found in the environment in higher concentrations than those established by Regulatory Organizations, as it was already mentioned.

The evaluation of phenol toxicity has become an area of active research. It had been studied on selected microorganisms (e.g. protozoa, yeast and bacteria), algae, duckweed and numerous invertebrates and vertebrates and varies widely with the organism tested, dissolved oxygen content and water temperature. It was observed that phenol induced teratogenic effect and depending on the organism tested, the acute toxicity estimated by the Media Lethal Concentration (LC50) value, varied from 6.5 to 1840 mg $L^{-1}$. Human consumption of phenol contaminated water can cause severe pain, blood changes, liver injury, muscular effects and even death. In addition, chronic toxic effects on human include vomiting, difficulty in swallowing, anorexia, liver and kidney damage, headache and other mental disturbances. It also induces hemolysis in human erythrocytes in vitro. The determination of urinary concentrations of phenols has been considered to be quite useful for the estimation of exposure, and its relationship with human diseases as well as laboratory abnormalities. Widespread human exposure to phenols has been documented recently and some of them, which are potential endocrine disruptors, have demonstrated adverse effects on male reproduction in animal and in vitro studies. The associations between human exposures to phenols on reproductive health are largely unknown. However, some researchers provide the first evidence that exposure to alkylphenols is associated with idiopathic male infertility. Due to the environmental problems related with the presence of phenolics in natural waters and soils, attempts have been focused on developing effective technologies for the removal of such compounds. Treatment systems generally only focus on the removal of regulated phenols such as phenol, 2,4-dichlorophenol (2,4-DCP) and pentachlorophenol (PCP) while the occurrence of un-regulated phenols in wastewater has not received sufficient attention. Nevertheless, many un-regulated phenols such as 4-t-octylphenol and 4-chloro-3- methylphenol are potentially hazardous to aquatic environments. Thus, the removal of both regulated and un-regulated phenolics is of considerable importance.

Numerous conventional physico-chemical methods based on the principles of adsorption, precipitation and coagulation, chemical oxidation, sedimentation, filtration, osmosis and ion exchange have been employed for the dephenolization of industrial wastewaters. Although several of these methods have demonstrated to be effective, most of them have several disadvantages such as high cost, incomplete purification and formation of hazardous byproducts; which limited their use. Thus, it has become necessary to look for environmentally friendly alternative technologies, such as biological methods, which are generally considered as safe and least disruptive treatments. These methods are based on the use of living organisms such as microorganisms like bacteria and fungi (bioremediation); algae (phycoremediation); terrestrial and aquatic plants (phytoremediation) and earthworms (vermiremediation) to manage or remediate polluted soils and water. All of them are well recognized as biotechnological tools to degrade or transformate contaminants into non- or less-toxic compounds. Generally, biological methods are cost-effective, environmentally sustainable and also socially acceptable. The present chapter focusses in bioremediation technologies for the treatment of water and effluents containing phenolics. In particular, phenol is taken as a representative toxic contaminant belonging to this class of compounds.

**Bacterial Phenol Bioremediation**

Biodegradation of phenol and metabolism as it was above mentioned, bioremediation is an innovative technology that involves the use of different microorganisms (bacteria and fungi) to remove, degrade or breakdown xenobiotic compounds in less toxic or non-toxic ones. However, this chapter will only emphasize on bacterial bioremediation. This technology includes different processes such as:

(a) Contaminant transformation,

(b) Degradation to simpler molecules,

(c) Mineralization into inorganic molecules such as $CO_2$, $H_2O$, $H_2$, $NH_3$, etc.,

(d) Sorption on cell surfaces and

(e) Intracellular accumulation, among others.

Some of these processes are mediated by enzymatic reactions that generate simpler compounds which enter into normal catabolic cell cycles. Since phenol is widespread in nature, bacteria capable of utilizing this compound as a carbon and energy source can be found in many different habitats. Several bacterial genera have been described as phenol degraders like Rhodococcus, Arthrobacter, Acinetobacter, Bacillus and Pseudomonas, among others. However, not all of them have developed adequate mechanisms to metabolize high phenol concentrations that can be found in anthropogenic sources such as industrial effluents. Moreover, there are many manmade phenol derivatives for which microorganism have not evolved degradation mechanisms, thus, these compounds persist in the environment as xenobiotics. The great potential of microorganisms to remediate phenolic compounds has motivated a number of studies focused on the elucidation of degradation process. Phenol degradation pathways under aerobic and anaerobic conditions Phenol metabolism can occur under aerobic ($O_2$ as electron acceptor) and/or anaerobic conditions ($NO_3^-$, $SO_4^{-2}$, $CO_2$ as final electron acceptors) although most research has been carried out on aerobic phenol degradation.

Under aerobic conditions, $O_2$ is a very important factor for hydroxylation and aromatic ring cleavage. In a first step, the enzyme phenol hydroxylase (a monoxygenase) which requires reduced pyrimidine nucleotide (NADH + $H^+$) adds a second hydroxyl group at the ortho position to the pre-existing hydroxyl group, to form catechol (1,2-dihydroxybenzene).

**Aerobic phenol biodegradation pathways proposed for bacterial strains**

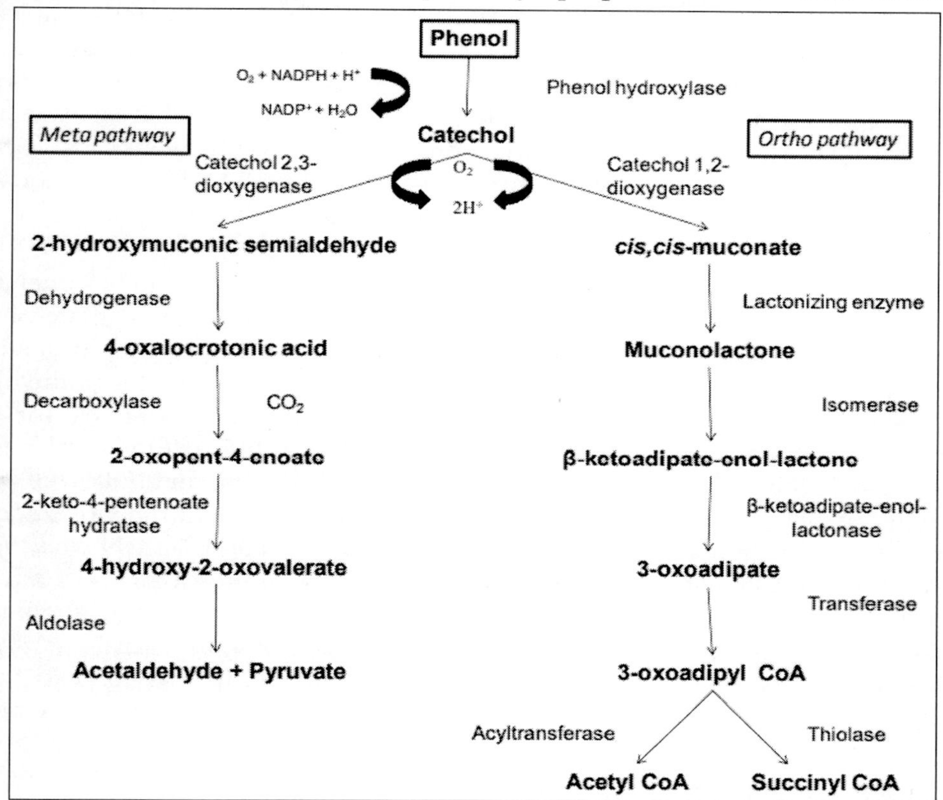


Regarding phenol hydroxylases, it has been described that they can be mono-component or multicomponent flavoproteins. In some species of Bacillus, Pseudomonas, Acinetobacter and Alcaligenes, phenol hydroxylases are mono-component, however, in *Acinetobacter radioresistens* and Pseudomonas sp. CF600, phenol hydroxylases are multicomponent. The formed catechol can be then degraded by dioxygenases through two different pathways, ortho or meta cleavage, depending on the involved microorganism. In the ortho- or β-ketoadipate pathway, the aromatic ring is cleaved between hydroxyl groups to form cis, cis-muconate, by a catechol 1,2-dioxygenase. This resulting compound is then metabolized to form acetyl CoA and succinyl-CoA, which are finally degraded in the Krebs cycle. Diverse bacteria are capable to degrade phenol by ortho- pathway, like *Acinetobacter calcoaceticus*, Pseudomonas species, Arthrobacter, Sphingomonas, Geobacillus and Rhodococcus. Regarding meta-pathway, the ring cleavage is catalyzed by the enzyme catechol 2,3- dioxygenase producing 2-hydroxymuconic semialdehyde. This product is finally transformed, after several reactions, in acetaldehyde and pyruvate, which are intermediates of the Krebs cycle. Researchers described that Pseudomonas putida, *P. cepacia, P. picketti* and *Alcaligenes eutrophus* metabolized phenol by meta-pathway. Comparing both pathways, ortho-pathway seems to be more efficient to convert carbon into biomass than meta-pathway, although phenol biodegradation process occurs at higher rate in bacteria that use meta-pathway. It is important to note that some bacterial strains were capable to degrade phenol through both pathways as it was described for Comamonas sp. and Cupriavidus sp. regarding to phenol anaerobic degradation, the knowledge is limited.

It has been established that anaerobic degradation includes phenol carboxilation in the para position to form 4-hydroxybenzoate, mediated by the enzyme 4-hydroxybenzoate carboxylase. Besides phenol, other aromatic compounds are also carboxylated as the first step of the anaerobic pathway. It was demonstrated for denitrifying Paracoccus, as well as for a methanogenic consortium capable to degrade catechol, ortho-cresol and ortho halogenated phenols, that they used para carboxylation, followed by dehydroxylation. Some microorganisms capable to degrade phenol under anaerobic conditions are *Desulphobacterium phenolicum* and *Thauera aromatic*. As it was previously described, both phenol degradation pathways have been thoroughly studied. Furthermore, the elucidation of the involved enzymes has recently allowed their use as molecular tools to estimate the diversity of phenol degrading bacterial communities. In this context, the coding gene for phenol hydroxylase and catechol 1,2 -dioxygenase enzymes have been applied with this purpouse.

**Phenol Bioremediation: *In vitro* Experiments**

In this section the focus will be put on in vitro experiments carried out to test optimal conditions for phenol removal from synthetic solutions that are generally performed before the scale-up in bioreactors.

There is an interesting review that collects studies related to microbial phenol biodegradation until the year 2006. It is clear from this work that Pseudomonas has been the most widely genus applied for the degradation of phenolic compounds as a single carbon and energy source. For example, it has been described that *P. putida* strains exhibit high degradation activity toward significant concentrations of phenol or its derivatives. In particular, the strain *P. putida* MTCC 1194 degraded 1000 mg $L^{-1}$ phenol after 162 h. Despite the significant amount of information gathered during the last years, phenol biodegradation is still an important challenge, which stimulates researchers to search new and more effective microbial species.

## Recently Studied Bacteria for Phenol Biodegradation

| Microorganisms | Isolation source | Maximum phenol concentration used (mg $L^{-1}$) |
|---|---|---|
| *Acinetobacter* sp.<br>*Comamonas* sp.<br>*Cupriavidus* sp.<br>*Pseudomonas* sp. | Natural soil | 180-900 |
| *Acinetobacter* sp. XA05 | Activated sludge | 1000 |
| *Rhodococcus coprophilus* | Semiarid soil | 800 |
| *Rhodococcus opacus lG* | ND | 750 |
| *Rhodococcus* sp. *UKM-P* | Oil contaminated soil | 500 |
| Consortium of 6 bacterial strains (*Bacillus* sp., *Arthrobacter* sp., *Halomonas* sp., *Pseudomonas* sp.) | Soil from saline environments | 300 |
| *Citrobacter freundi*<br>*Proteus mirabilis* | Oil contaminated soil | 100 |
| *Pseudomonas* sp. *a3* | Activated sludge | 100 |
| *Acinetohacter* sp. EBRO1<br>*Actnetobacter* sp. EBR02<br>*Cobetia marina* EBR04 | Intestine of marine creatures | 100 |
| *Ralstonia pickettii* | Petroleum refinery oil sludge | 200 |
| *Rhodococcus* sp. *CSl* | Tannery effluent | 1000 |
| *Planococcus sp. S5* | Activated sludge | 380 |
| *Acinetobacter* sp. RTEJ1.4 | Industrial effluent | 600 |
| *Rhodococcus* sp. *UKMP-5M* | Oil contaminated soil | 1000 |
| *Rhodococcus* sp. *AQ5NOL 2* | Contaminated soil | 500 |
| *Bacillus cereus WJ1* | Contaminated wastewater | 600 |

It is noteworthy, from this Table, that the focus of these works was the isolation and characterization of native phenol degrading bacterial strains from highly polluted sites and the optimization of culture conditions to maximize the biodegradation process (pH, temperature, initial phenol concentrations, agitation and presence of different nutrients, among others). Moreover, in some of them the presence and activity of key enzymes are described. It is important to note that 1000 mg $L^{-1}$ appears to be the maximum concentration of phenol used in these experiments. At higher phenol concentration microorganisms suffer from substrate inhibition, by which the growth is inhibited and hence phenol is not degraded. For this reason, new developments to improve biodegradation are being performed including the use of bacterial consortia, immobilized cells on different natural or synthetic materials and co-metabolism of phenol with another substrate, among others.

## Bacterial Immobilization as a useful Strategy for an Efficient Phenol Biodegradation

As it was pointed out before, the use of free bacteria strains for bioremediation purposes has been well documented. However, the immobilization of bacterial cells has given some advantages to the process such as: greater active biomass availability, greater resistance to high toxic compound concentrations, increase of catalytic activity and the alternative of reusing the immobilized cells for consecutive biodegradation cycles. In particular, for phenol biodegradation, the immobilization of bacterial biomass is an effective technique to protect bacteria from high concentrations of this compound. With this purpose, cells immobilized in different support matrices such as polyacrylamide, polyvinyl alcohol (PVA), agar, agarose, polysulphone, polyacrylnitrile, calcium alginate (Ca-alginate) and others have been used with different results. There are many evidences about the reduction of the toxicity of high phenol concentrations (considered as bactericides for free cells) and hence a higher degradative ability when bacteria are immobilized on Ca-alginate. This increase in the efficiency was explained not only by higher reaction ability due to the high density of immobilized cells, but also by a protective effect of the polymer giving a more favorable microenvironment for the catalytic reaction. Two Ca-alginate immobilized Bacillus cereus strains showed higher phenol degradation efficiency than free cells at high phenol concentrations (1500-2000 mg $L^{-1}$), indicating the improved tolerance of the immobilized cells toward phenol toxicity. Besides, these immobilized cells were able to degrade more than 50% of 2000 mg $L^{-1}$ phenol within 26 and 36 d. However, there are some reports which showed better rates and efficiencies for phenol degradation using Ca-alginate immobilized cells. For example, researchers found that *P. aeruginosa* cells immobilized in Ca-alginate were able to completely degrade 900 and 1200 mg $L^{-1}$ of phenol after 80 and 290 h, respectively.

### Examples of Immobilized Bacterial Cells in different Support Matrices used for Biodegradation of Phenols

| Immobilized bacterial species | Immobilization matrix | Phenol concentration (mg $L^{-1}$) | Time required for degradation |
|---|---|---|---|
| (1) | (2) | (3) | (4) |
| *Bacillus cereus* strains AKG 1 and AKG 2 | Ca-alginate | 2000 | 26-36 days (50%) |
| *Pseudomonas aeniginosa* | Ca-alginate | 900<br>1200 | 80 h (100%)<br>290 h (100%) |
| *Acinetobacter and Sphingomonas* | PYA | 800 | 35 h (100%) |

*(Contd...)*

| (1) | (2) | (3) | (4) |
|---|---|---|---|
| *Acinetobacter* sp. strain PDI2 | PYA | 500 | 9 h (100%) |
| *Pseudomonas* sp. SAO1 | Alginate<br>Pectin<br>PVA-alginate<br>Glycerol-alginate<br>ACA | 2000 | PVA-alginate 100 h (100%)<br>ACA 110 h (100%) |
| Enriched microorganisms from a compost of agricultural wastes | AC-alginate<br>AC-clay-alginate | 1630 | 38 h (90%)<br>44 h (100%) |

Other essential factors for practical application of Ca-alginate immobilized cells are the optimization of the polymer percentage in the beads, reusability and stability during longterm storage. The increase of Ca-alginate percentage (2-5%) in the beads affects negatively the degradation rate of contaminants, which could be explained by a lower diffusion of oxygen, nutrients and even the substrate into the beads, as it was demonstrated by several researchers. Many authors evaluate the stability of the bacterial immobilized cells after long periods of time, varying from months to years, in order to propose the strategy as a cost effective and economically viable process for bioremediation. Different polymer types and combinations for cell immobilization were used for phenol removal assays and the results were compared. In this sense, it has been found that Pseudomonas cells immobilized on either Ca-alginate beads, combined beads of PVAalginate or alginate-chitosan-alginate (ACA) capsules resulted in remarkable reduction (65%) in phenol degradation time compared to free cells. Among them, cells immobilized on PVAalginate and ACA provided the best performance for high phenol concentrations, producing complete degradation of 2000 mg $L^{-1}$ phenol after 100 and 110 h, respectively. Also, the effect of activated carbon (AC) and clay addition to alginate beads was studied and the performance for phenol biodegradation of the immobilized cells was compared. These authors deepened about the diffusive mass transfer within the solid matrix and they found a notorious limitation of diffusion when the matrix contained clay and AC in alginate beads; however this combination contributed to better mineralization of phenol at high concentrations. As it was mentioned before, the PVA has also been used for cell immobilization. In this sense, mixed cells of Acinetobacter and Sphingomonas immobilized in PVA exhibited higher degradation rate than free cells for phenol concentrations from 500 to 1000 mg $L^{-1}$, even in a broader range of pH and temperatures. However, there is a main drawback with the entrapment immobilization technique using PVA because it includes a step during which bacteria are exposed to sub-freezing temperatures during the cross linking stage.

For this reason, researchers modified some steps of immobilization avoiding chilling temperatures, in order to extend the application of PVA-immobilization to other bacterial genera. However, some bacterial strains like *P. putida* are not affected by the freezing step. Actually, there is an increasing search for low-cost, more efficient and easier to handle support matrices. Thus, different residual products have been used to immobilize cells, such as tubings, packed columns, granulated activated carbon, coconut shells, etc. In this context, Robledo Ortíz *et al*., (2010) proposed and thoroughly studied the adhesion property of bacteria to fiber-polymer foamed composites produced from waste materials like recycled polyethylene and agave fiber from *Agave tequilana*, a plant used for tequila production. For phenol biodegradation, *P. putida* cells have been immobilized in activated pumice particles. On the other hand, Del Castillo *et al*. (2012) found that several (chloro) phenol degrading bacteria were able to colonize the surface of cork particles in the presence of phenol. For this reason, the authors proposed that bacterial immobilization on these particles would be a valuable tool to perform the self-remediation of wastewaters derived of cork processing. Other cost effective and environmental friendly matrices have been proved for bacterial immobilization such as linen shells, an abundantly available agro-waste, or a natural fibrous material obtained from the mature dried fruits of *Luffa cylindrica* L., which could be ideal alternatives to the expensive solid matrices for the development of bioremediation processes and other biotechnological applications. Possibly, in the following years, new alternative matrices derived from residual materials would become useful for immobilization process, contributing with the disposal of great volumes of wastes. Another important aspect that is gaining attention within the scientific community for an efficient bioremediation process is the design and improvement of different types of bioreactors with free and immobilized cells, as it will be described in the following section.

**Use of Bioreactors for Phenol Biodegradation**

Current technology for biodegradation of toxic compounds, including phenols, involves the use of bioreactors, in batch and continuous processes, using either free or immobilized cells. Bioreactors are generally defined as devices in which biological and/or biochemical processes are developed under closely monitored and tightly controlled environmental and operating conditions (e.g. pH, temperature, pressure, nutrient supply and agitation). The high degree of reproducibility, low contamination risk, control and automatization introduced by bioreactors for specific experimental bioprocesses has been key for their transfer to largescale applications, including its use for wastewater treatments. In the case of wastewater containing phenol, its treatment has been focused on employing and exploring new types of bioreactors with high performance for practical utilization. These include the use of hollow fiber membrane contactors, fluidized bed bioreactor, microbial fuel cells system and fixed-biofilm process. Other novel bioreactors that have been developed for bio-treatment applications include rotating rope bioreactor, two phase partitioning bioreactors (TPPBs) and foam emulsion bioreactor. It is important to note that although bio-treatment schemes using bioreactors are based on aerobic, anaerobic and combined aerobic-anaerobic processes, the focus in this section will be put on the aerobic ones.

**Anaerobic Phenol Biodegradation Pathway proposed for Bacterial Strains**

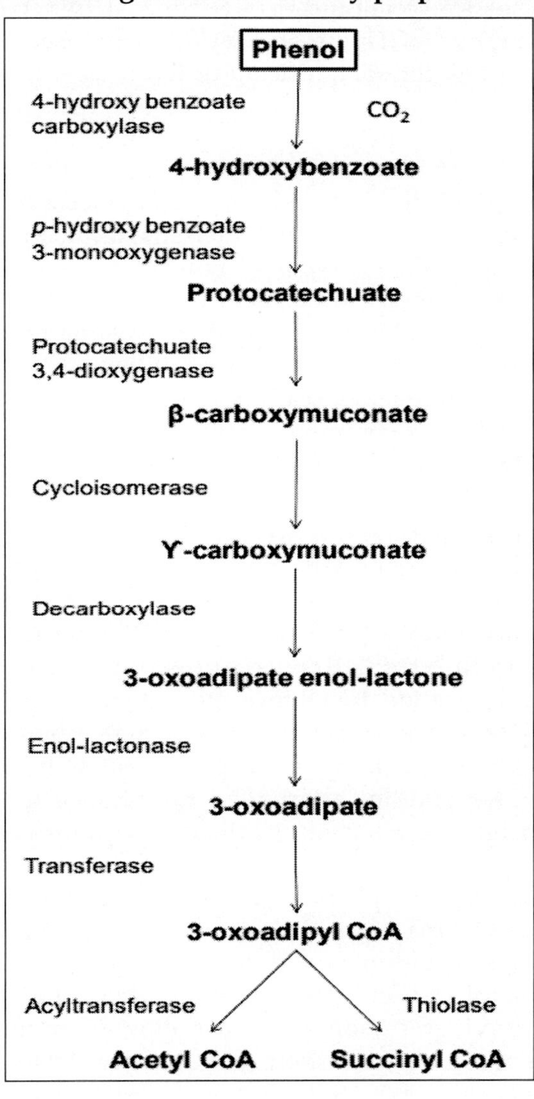

It is noteworthy that the overall efficiency of the bacterial biomass in the biodegradation of phenol may be affected by many factors such as phenol concentration, temperature, the presence of other nutrients, the presence of other pollutants and bacterial density. In this sense, El-Naas, Al Muhtaseb and Makhlouf (2009) demonstrated that the biodegradation capabilities of *P. putida* were highly affected by temperature, pH, initial phenol concentration and the biomass density in a bubble column bioreactor. Furthermore, optimization of aeration is another essential aspect in order to maximize phenol removal efficiency in a bioreactor. Paisio *et al.* (2012) also evaluated the effect of aeration and agitation on growth and phenol removal efficiency of Rhodococcus sp. CS1 in a stirred tank bioreactor. In this study, when aeration of 1 vvm and 3 vvm were used, complete phenol removal was observed without significant differences between two agitation rates used (200 and 400 rpm). In contrast, at 600 rpm of agitation and 3 vvm of aeration, only 38% of phenol removal and a lower biomass were observed, compared with aeration of 1 vvm. This result could indicate that high aeration and agitation produced stress in bacteria and probably may result in cell rupture, which inhibited their metabolism and growth and consequently decreased phenol removal efficiency. Due to the advantages of immobilized bacterial cells, they have been used in combination with bioreactors. In this sense, Aneez Ahamad and Mohammad Kunhi (2011) compared the performance of free and immobilized cells of Pseudomonas CP4 in a fluidized bed bioreactor. In batch runs, with an aeration rate of 1 vvm, at 30°C and pH 7.0 agar immobilized cells degraded up to 3000 mg L-1 of phenol as compared to 1500 mg L-1 by Ca-alginate immobilized cells whereas free cells could degrade only 1000 mg $L^{-1}$.

In a continuous process with Ca-alginate immobilized cells a degradation rate of 200 mg L -1 h -1 was obtained while agar-entrapped cells were better since they could withstand and degrade up to 4000 mg L -1 phenol with a maximum degradation rate of 400 mg L-1 h -1. In another study, Al-Zuhair and El-Nass (2011), using two types of bioreactors namely bubble column and spouted bed bioreactor, demonstrated that *P. putida* immobilized on PVA particles could remove high phenol concentrations and that bacteria remained active for a period of 72 h, even without the addition of nutrients. Another alternative to enhance the biodegradation of the pollutant in bioreactors can be called a cooperative phenol removal system between biological and physical treatment. In this process adsorption plays a key role in decreasing phenol concentration during adaptation period at which microorganisms cannot degrade phenol, avoiding substrate inhibition. After the adaptation period, the microorganism starts to degrade the remaining phenol concentration. For example, Li and Wang (2008) enhanced phenol biodegradation using a hollow-fiber membrane, by the addition of granular activated carbon (GAC) (hybrid bioreactor). In batch biotransformation experiments, complete removal of 1000 mg $L^{-1}$ phenol (concentration at which free cells cannot grow) was accomplished within 18 h in the hybrid bioreactor, comparing with 23 h in the GAC free bioreactor. At continuous running, the GAC bioreactor showed its superiority over the GAC free bioreactor during start-up and elevated loading phase. More than 90% of phenol was transformed in the GAC bioreactor when the phenol loading was < 24 mg $h^{-1}$. The authors concluded that the better bioreactor performance may be due to the enhanced mass transportation and adsorption capacity with the incorporation of GAC. Kwon, Jung & Yeom (2009) found that a porous polymer bead of PVA and Xanthan gum was the best entrapment for phenol degradation by *P. fluorescens* KNU417. Besides, when AC (1%) was co-immobilized with microorganisms in the bead, the start-up period was shortened by 40 h and the removal efficiency of phenol during the period was increased by 28% than beads containing only microorganisms.

On the other hand, Zhao *et al.* (2009) used organic modified montmorillonite (OMMT) as delivery agents for phenol to microorganisms in TPPBs (OMMT-PSF) and polyurethane foam immobilized microorganisms (PUF-immobilized microorganisms) as biocatalysts. Phenol biodegradation rates of batch fermentation were examined, concluding that the maximum volumetric consumption rate of phenol decreased in the order: immobilized microorganisms with OMMT-PSF capsules (342.4 mg $L^{-1}$ $h^{-1}$) > immobilized microorganisms without OMMT-PSF capsules (300 mg $L^{-1}$ $h^{-1}$) > free microorganisms with OMMT-PSF capsules (208.4 mg $L^{-1}$ $h^{-1}$) > free microorganisms without OMMT-PSF capsules (125.8 mg $L^{-1}$ $h^{-1}$). These results demonstrated that the use of immobilized microorganisms and OMMT-PSF capsules in TPPB offers improved degradation of phenol. Finally, the choice of the most suitable bioreactor will be determined by many factors including the scale, the method of aeration, the mixing mechanism and the resistance of the cells to the shear stress generated in the bioreactor. At last, all of these factors will determine the biodegradation capabilities. In addition, bioreactor-based technology allows the management of high volumes and degradation of toxic compounds commonly found in industrial effluents.

**Biodegradation of Phenolic Compounds from Industrial Wastewaters**

Industrial effluents can contain different organic and/or inorganic contaminants, therefore their bioremediation represent an important challenge. As it was previously mentioned, biological treatments using both anaerobic and aerobic systems have been recognized as effective methods for the degradation of highly polluted industrial wastewaters, including those containing different phenolic compounds. Bio-treatments can be performed at different scales such as Erlenmeyers flasks, bioreactors of variable volume as well as pilot-scale experiments. Most of the studies in this field employ chemical or biological oxygen demand (COD/BOD) determinations as indicators of bioremediation. In addition, the removal of phenolic compounds is also evaluated in some effluents such as those derived from olive oil extraction, paper factories, tanneries, crude oil refineries, palm oil and phenolic resin producing industries and coke and coal gasification processes.

**A brief Summary of recent Research Studies on Bacterial Wastewater Bioremediation**

| Wastewater | Phenols concentration (mg $L^{-1}$) | Microorganisms |
|---|---|---|
| Olive mill extraction | Phenol (1200) | Mixed culture |
| | Phenols (4300) | Actived sludge |
| Paper factory | Phenols (364) | Mixed culture |
| | Chlorophenol (82)/PCP (100) | *Pseudomonas stutzeri* CL7 |
| Tannery | Phenols (17.5) | *Rhodococcus* sp. CSI |
| Petroleum refinery | Phenol (637) | *Pseudomonas* sp. PD39 |
| Phenolic resin manufacture | Phenol (250-4000) | Nitrifying and heterotrophic bacteria |
| POME | Phenols (33.6) | *Lactobacillus plantarum* SF5 |
| | Phenol (100-1000) | *Thermoanaerobacterium*-rich sludge |
| Coal gasification | Phenols (342-487) | Actived sludge |

This is important considering that olive oil extraction is one of the activities that generate great quantities of highly toxic phenolic wastes. Omer (2012) indicated that the phenol content (1200 mg $L^{-1}$ ) of olive mill wastewater gradually decreased reaching the maximum removal (71.9 and 71.4%) after 25 days of treatment using a bacterial mixture constituted by *Azotobacter vinelandii, P. putida* and *P. fluorescens*, grown at 50 and 30% of effluent dilution, respectively. In addition, Gonçalves *et al.* (2012) also observed remarkable phenols removal efficiencies (up 60%) in up-flow anaerobic reactors, inoculated with active sludge, which were intermittently feeded with raw olive mill wastewater containing 4300 mg $L^{-1}$ of phenols. Khoufi, Aloui and Sayadi (2009) described a novel process developed at pilot scale for the treatment of olive mill wastewater, which combines electro-Fenton, anaerobic digestion and ultrafiltration. Application of these procedures allowed obtaining high removal efficiencies of phenolic compounds (95% of initial concentration of 1150 mg $L^{-1}$). This work remarks the need of integrating physico-chemical treatments and biological processes for the degradation of recalcitrant compounds, as it was previously indicated by other researchers. The efficiency of bacteria for phenolic compounds removal from paper factory effluents has been extensively studied. Recently, Chandra and Singh (2012) demonstrated that a mixed culture constituted by *Pseudochrobactrum glaciale* IITRP1, *Providencia rettgeri* IITRP2 and Pantoea sp RCT2 degraded 61% and 90% of total phenols and chlorophenol from pulp paper mill effluent containing initial concentrations of 364 and 82 mg $L^{-1}$, respectively, within 216 h.

Other authors have also evaluated PCP degradation in these effluents. Regarding this, Singh *et al.* (2008) studied a mixed culture of two bacterial strains, Bacillus sp. and *Serratia marcescens*, which was able to degrade up to 94% of the PCP present in a pulp paper mill effluent at initial concentration of 1440 mg L -1 after 168 h. Moreover, Karn, Chakrabarty and Reddy (2010) demonstrated that P. stutzeri strain CL7 was able to remove 66.8% of PCP from the secondary sludge of pulp and paper mill supplemented with 100 mg $L^{-1}$ of PCP after two weeks. Nair, Jayachandran and Shashidhar (2007) used free and immobilized cells of Alcaligenes sp. D (2) in a packed bed reactor to treat a paper factory effluent containing 9.41 mg $L^{-1}$ of phenol. Both cells removed a maximum of 99% of phenol after 20 h of treatment using a batch process. In the continuous mode of operation the strain was able to achieve 99% phenol removal. A combined chemical/biological process for the treatment of paper mill effluent (activated sludge-ozonation processes) was described. The combined activated sludge-$O_3$/pH 10 treatment was able to remove around 70 % of total phenols (initial concentration of 10-30 mg $L^{-1}$). Tannery wastewater usually contains high concentrations of organic matter, including phenols and other chemicals. These effluents cannot be released into the environment without pre-treatment because of their high toxicity. Thus, in recent years the efficiency of several bacterial strains for treating tannery wastewater has been studied. For instance, Paisio *et al.* (2012) observed that Rhodococcus sp. CS1 strain was able to grow and completely degrade phenols from tannery effluents containing 17.5 mg $L^{-1}$ of total phenols, after 9 h of incubation. Srivastava, Ahmad and Thakur (2007) studied PCP biodegradation in a sequential bioreactor and determined that tannery effluents treated initially by bacterial consortium followed by the fungus *Aspergillus niger* FK1 removed 67% of PCP, whereas in another set of bioreactor in which effluents were treated initially by fungi followed by bacteria could remove 58% of PCP. Chandra *et al.* (2011) evaluated the tannery wastewater bioremediation in aeration lagoons at a common effluent treatment plant from Uttar Pradesh, India. Most of the organic pollutants detected in the tannery wastewaters were diminished and 77% reduction of phenolics was obtained by bacterial treatment. Reports on petroleum refinery effluents biotreatment are relatively abundant in the literature. However, only few of them describe the biodegradation of phenols. This is an important feature to take into account because high phenolics contents have been found in these wastewaters (up to 2000 mg $L^{-1}$), as it was previously mentioned. In this sense, Ojumu *et al.* (2005) studied the ability of *P. aeruginosa* and *P. fluorescens* strains for phenol biodegradation from refinery effluent, in a batch reactor. Phenol (30 mg $L^{-1}$) was degraded completely by both bacterial species after 60 and 84 h, respectively. Subsequently, Bako *et al.* (2008) studied mixed cultures of *P. aeruginosa* and *Penicillium janthinellum*. These microorganisms removed 50-100 % phenol (1.48-3.10 mg $L^{-1}$) from effluents of a refinery of crude oil after two weeks of incubation. Better results were achieved by Ren *et al.* (2008) using Pseudomonas sp. PD39, that was capable to remove 637 mg $L^{-1}$ of phenol from wastewaters of a petroleum chemical plant only in 72 h.

Similarly to the petroleum refinery effluents, few research studies showing the bacterial phenolics biodegradation from wastewaters derived from phenolic resin industries have been published. Among them, Eiroa *et al.* (2008) showed that phenol (250-4000 mg $L^{-1}$) from this wastewater was completely removed at all concentrations combining nitrifying bacteria, contained in an anoxic reactor, with heterotrophic bacteria of an aerobic reactor. These results are promising taking into account the high phenol concentrations detected and removed from these wastewaters. Another understudied area is the bio-treatment of phenols contained in palm oil mill effluent (POME). POME is a highly polluted wastewater exhibiting high COD, BOD and phenol concentration. Limkhuansuwan and Chaiprasert (2010) demonstrated that *Lactobacillus plantarum* SF5 removed 34% of phenolic compounds (33.6 mg $L^{-1}$) contained in POME. More recently, Mamimin *et al.* (2012), used a Thermoanaero bacterium-rich sludge for hydrogen production and phenol removal from POME in the presence of phenol concentrations from 100 to 1000 mg $L^{-1}$, obtaining high removal efficiencies (up to 92%). Conventional biological processes do not always provide satisfactory results for industrial wastewater treatment, since many of the organic substances produced by chemical industries are toxic or resistant to biological treatment.

In this context, some inhibitory effects of coke and coal gasification wastewaters on different microorganisms were observed. For example, Cordova-Rosa *et al.* (2009) observed that an indigenous bacterial consortium as well as a pure culture of *Acinetobacter calcoaceticus* var. anitratus growing in coke gasification wastewater, were inhibited and no phenol biodegradation was observed after 10 days of incubation. Similarly, direct biological treatment of coke factory wastewaters by a consortium of Chlorella vulgaris strain and Alcaligenes sp. was not possible due to the toxicity of organic compounds. However, complete phenol degradation was achieved when the effluent was pre-treated with activated carbon adsorption and UV(A-B)-irradiation, demonstrating the importance of combined physicochemical and biological tools. On the other hand, Li *et al.* (2011) also obtained promising results using a laboratory-scale moving bed biofilm reactor (MBBR) to study the biodegradation of coal gasification wastewater by an acclimated activated sludge. Maximum removal efficiencies of 89% were obtained for phenols after 12 d. Bioremediation of phenolics in other wastewaters from textiles or pharmaceuticals industries and explosives, dyes or cumene manufacture is an area less explored. Therefore, it requires to be more studied.

## CONCLUSION

As it was highlighted in this project report, the application of bacteria for phenol bioremediation is a promising technology that is being continuously improved. Several bacterial genera have demonstrated to be efficient for phenol removal from wastewaters. Moreover, mixed bacterial cultures sometimes offer more advantages because they can better withstand different environmental conditions. Although an extensive knowledge is now available in this regard, the appropriate and continuous selection of more efficient microorganisms is still an area of great interest. In order to implement an efficient bioremediation technology, a scientific and well formulated strategy must be carried out taking into consideration several aspects that influence the process. In this sense, immobilization is an effective methodology to protect bacteria from high concentrations of toxic compounds, and also allow reusing and stability during long-term storage. These properties are essential factors for practical application of immobilized cells for bioremediation. The search of new and low-cost matrices would be useful to make this process more economical- and environmentally viable. Moreover, combination of immobilization with the design and use of proper bioreactors would confer several advantages to optimize and improve phenol removal of great volumes of contaminated solutions and/or effluents. Nevertheless, additional basic research, such as toxicity studies of the formed metabolites is of concern and need further investigation to apply this technology in a safe way. In addition, the use of the currently emergingomic approaches (genomics, metagenomics, proteomics, metabolomics, etc.) applied in a novel and imaginative way could allow to understand interesting aspects of the complex biodegradation pathways and, therefore, they can be used to enhance phenol remediation applicability. It is expected that a combined approach, integrating recent findings and using different strategies simultaneously, could be used to successfully improve the efficiency of phenol bioremediation, allowing the application of this technology in a large scale which is one of the most important challenges from an environmental point of view.

## REFERENCES

1. Agarry, S.E. and Salomon, B.O. (2008). Kinetics of Batch Microbial Degradation of Phenols by Indigenous *Pseudomonas fluorescens*. Int. J. Environ. Sci. Technol. 5, 223-232.

2. Agarry, S.E., Solomon, B.O. and Layokun, S.K. (2008). Kinetics of Batch Microbial Degradation of Phenols by Indigenous Binary mixed Culture of Pseudomonas Aeruginosa and Pseudomonas Fluorescence. African J. Biotechnol. 7, 2417-2423.
3. Aksu, Z. (2005). Application of Biosorption for the Removal of Organic Pollutants: A Review. Process Biochem. 40, 997-1026.
4. Al-Zuhair S. and El-Naas M.H. (2011). Immobilization of *Pseudomonas putida* in PVA gel Particles for the Biodegradation of Phenol at High Concentrations. Biochem. Eng. J. 56, 46-50.
5. Al-Zuhair, S. and El-Naas, M.H. (2012). Phenol Biodegradation by *Ralstonia pickettii* Extracted from Petroleum Refinery Oil Sludge. Chem. Eng. Commun. 199 (9), 1194-1204.
6. Amuda, O.S. and Ibrahim, A.O. (2006). Industrial Wastewater Treatment using Natural Material as Adsorbent. African J. Biotechnol. 5(16), 1483-1487.
7. Aneez Ahamad, P.Y. and Mohammad Kunhi, A.A. (2011). Enhanced Degradation of Phenol by Pseudomonas sp. CP4 Entrapped in Agar and Calcium Alginate Beads in Batch and Continuous Processes. Biodegradation 22, 253-265.
8. Arif, N.M., Ahmad, S.A., Syed, M.A. and Shukor, M.Y. (2013). Isolation and Characterization of a Phenol-degrading Rhodococcus sp. strain AQ5NOL 2 KCTC 11961BP. J. Basic Microbiol. 53(1), 9-19.
9. Assalin, M.R., Dos Santos Almeida, E. and Durán, N. (2009). Combined System of Activated Sludge and Ozonation for the Treatment of Kraft E1 Effluent. Int. J. Environ. Res. Public Health 6(3), 1145-1154.
10. Bajza, Z. and Vrcek, I.V. (2001). Water Quality Analysis of Mixtures Obtained from Tannery Waste Effluents. Ecotoxicol. Environ. Saf. 50(1), 15-18.
11. Bako, S.P., Chukwunonso, D. and Adamu, A.K. (2008). Bio-remediation of Refinery Effluents by Strains of *Pseudomonas aeruginosa* and *Penicillium janthinellum*. Appl. Ecol. Environ. Res. 6(3), 49-60.
12. Banerjee, A. and Ghoshal, A.K. (2011). Phenol Degradation Performance by Isolated Bacillus cereus Immobilized in Alginate. Int. Biodet. Biodeg. 65, 1052-1060.
13. Basile, L.A. and Erijman, L. (2008). Quantitative Assessment of Phenol Hydroxylase Diversity in Bioreactors using Functional Gene Analysis. Appl. Microbiol. Biotechnol. 78, 863-872.
14. Basu, S.K., Oleszkiewicz, J.A. and Sparling, R. (1996). Dehalogenation of 2-chlorophenol (2- CP) in Anaerobic batch Cultures. Water Res. 30, 315-322.
15. Behera, S., Mohanty, R.C. and Ray, R.C. (2012). Ethanol Fermentation of Sugarcane Molasses by Zymomonas Mobilis MTCC 92 Immobilized in Luffa cylindrical L. sponge discs and Caalginate matrices. Braz. J. Microbiol. 43(4), 1499-1507.
16. Bernadini, G., Spinelli, O., Presutti, C., Vismara, C., Bolzacchini, E., Orlando, M. and Settimi, R. (1996). Evaluation of the Developmental Toxicity of Pesticide MCPA and its Contaminants Phenol and Chlorocresol. Environ. Toxicol. Chem. 15, 754-760.
17. Bukowska, B. and Kowalska, S. (2004). Phenol and Catechol Induce Prehemolytic and Haemolytic changes in Human Erythrocytes. Toxicol. Lett. 152, 73-84.
18. Carvalho, M.F., Vasconcelos, I., Bull, A.T. and Castro, P.M.L. (2001). A GAC Biofilm Reactor for the Continuous Degradation of 4-chlorophenol: Treatment Efficiency and Microbial Analysis. Appl. Microbiol. Biotechnol. 57, 419-426.
19. Chakraborty, S., Bhattacharya, T., Patel, T.N. and Tiwari, K.K. (2010). Biodegradation of Phenol by Native Microorganisms Isolated from Coke Processing Wastewater. J. Environ. Biol. 31, 293-296.

20. Chandra, R., Bharagava, R.N., Kapley, A. and Purohit, H.J. (2011). Bacterial Diversity, Organic Pollutants and their Metabolites in Two Aeration Lagoons of Common Effluent Treatment Plant (CETP) during the Degradation and Detoxification of Tannery Wastewater. Biores. Technol. 102, 2333-2341.
21. Chandra, R. and Singh, R. (2012). Decolourisation and Detoxification of Rayon Grade Pulp Paper Mill Effluent by Mixed Bacterial Culture Isolated from Pulp Paper Mill Effluent Polluted Site. Biochem. Eng. J. 61, 49-58.
22. Chang, C.C., Tseng, S.K., Chang, C.C. and Ho, C.M. (2003). Reductive Dechlorination of 2- chlorophenol in a Hydrogenotrophic, Gas Permeable, Silicone Membrane Bioreactor. Biores. Technol. 90, 323-328.
23. Chen, M., Tang, R., Fu, G., Xu, B., Zhu, P., Qiao, S., Chen, X., Xu, B., Qin, Y., Lu, C., Hang, B., Xia, Y. and Wang, X. (2013). Association of Exposure to Phenols and Idiopathic Male Infertility. J. Hazard. Mater. (250-251), 115-121.
24. Chen, Y., Hong, L., Han, W., Wang, L., Sun, X. and Li, J. (2011). Treatment of High Explosive Production Wastewater Containing RDX by Combined Electrocatalytic Reaction and Anoxic-oxic Biodegradation. Chem. Eng. J. 168(3), 1256-1262.
25. Cordova-Rosa, S.M., Dams, R.I., Cordova-Rosa, E.V., Radetski, M.R., Corrêa, A.X.R. and Radetski, C.M. (2009). Remediation of Phenol-contaminated Soil by a Bacterial Consortium and *Acinetobacter calcoaceticus* Isolated from an Industrial Wastewater Treatment Plant. J. Hazard. Mater. 164(1), 61-66.
26. Del Castillo, I., Hernández, P., Lafuente, A., Rodríguez-Llorente, I.D., Caviedes, M.A. and Pajuelo E. (2012). Self-bioremediation of Cork-processing Wastewaters by (chloro) Phenoldegrading Bacteria Immobilised onto Residual Cork Particles. Water Res. 46, 1723-1734.
27. Della Greca, M., Monaco, P., Pinto, G., Pollio, A., Previtera, L. and Temussi, F., (2001). Phytotoxicity of Low-molecular-weight Phenols from Olive Mill Waste Waters. Bull. Environ. Contam. Toxicol. 67(3), 352-359.
28. Diya'uddeen, B.H., Wan Daud, W.M.A. and Abdul Aziz, A.R. (2011). Treatment Technologies for Petroleum Refinery Effluents: A Review. Process Saf. Environ. Protec. 89(2), 95-105.
29. Eiroa, M., Vilar, A., Kennes, C. and Veiga, M.C. (2008). Effect of Phenol on the Biological Treatment of Wastewaters from a Resin Producing Industry. Biores. Technol. 99(9), 3507-3512.
30. Eker, S. and Kargi, F. (2008). COD, 2,4,6-trichlorophenol (TCP) and Toxicity Removal from Synthetic Wastewater in Rotating Perforated-tubes Biofilm Reactor. J. Hazard. Mater. 159(2-3), 306-312.
31. El Azhari, N., Devers-Lamrani, M.C., Guillaume, R., Nadine, M. and Laurent, F. (2010). Molecular analysis of the Catechol-degrading Bacterial Community in a Coal Wasteland Heavily Contaminated with PAHs. J. Hazard. Mater. 177(1-3), 593-601.
32. El-Naas, M.H., Al-Muhtaseb, S.A. and Makhlouf, S. (2010a). Batch Degradation of Phenol in a Spouted Bed Bioreactor System. J. Indust. Eng. Chem. 16, 267-272.
33. El-Naas, M.H., Al-Zuhair, S. and Makhlouf, S. (2010b). Continuous Biodegradation of Phenol in a Spouted Bed Bioreactor (SBBR). Chem. Eng. J. 160, 565-570.
34. El-Naas, M.H., Al-Muhtaseb, S.A. and Makhlouf, S. (2009). Biodegradation of Phenol by Pseudomonas putida Immobilized in Polyvinyl Alcohol (PVA) gel. J. Hazard. Mater. 164, 720-725.
35. El-Sayed, W., Ibrahim, M., Abu-Shady, M., El-Beih, F., Ohmura, N., Saiki, H. and Ando, A. (2003). Isolation and Characterization of Phenol-degrading Bacteria from a Coking Plant. Biosci. Biotechnol. Biochem. 67(9), 2026-2029.

36. Essam, T., Amin, M.A., El Tayeb, O., Mattiasson, B. and Guieysse, B. (2006). Biological Treatment of Industrial Wastes in a Photobioreactor. Water Sci. Technol. 53(11), 117-125.
37. Farrell, A. and Quilty, B. (2002). The Enhancement of 2-chlorophenol Degradation by a mixed Microbial Community when Augmented with Pseudomonas putida CP1. Water Res. 36, 2443- 2450.
38. Field, J.A. and Sierra-Alvarez, R. (2008). Microbial Degradation of Chlorinated Phenols. Rev. Environ. Sci. Biotechnol. 7, 211-241.
39. Flocco, C.G., Lo Balbo, A., Carranza, M.P. and Giulietti, A.M. (2002). Removal of Phenol by Alfalfa Plants (Medicago sativa L.) Grown in Hydroponics and its Effect on some Physiological Parameters. Acta Biotechnol. 22, 43-54.
40. Gayathri, V.K. and Vasudevan, N. (2010). Enrichement of Phenol Degrading Moderately Halophilic Bacterial Consortium from Saline. J. Biorem. Biodeg. 1(1), 1-6.
41. Gonçalves, M.R., Costa, J.C., Marques, I.P. and Alves, M.M. (2012). Strategies for Lipids and Phenolics Degradation in the Anaerobic Treatment of Olive Mill Wastewater. Water Res. 46(6), 1684-1692.
42. Gouda, M.K. (2007). Immobilization of Rhodococcus sp. DG for Efficient Degradation of Phenol. Fresen. Environ. Bull. 16(12b), 1655-1661.
43. Guzik, U., Greñ, I., Hupert-Kocurek, K. and Wojcieszyñka, D. (2011). Catechol 1,2-dioxygenase from the New Aromatic Compounds-degrading *Pseudomonas putida* Strain N6. Int. Biodet. Biodeg. 65, 504-512.
44. Harrison, M.A.J., Barra, S., Borghesi, D., Vione, D., Arsene C. and Olariu, R.I. (2005). Nitrated Phenols in the Atmosphere: A Review. Atmospheric Environ. 39, 231-248.
45. Harwood, C.S. and Parales, R.E. (1996). The β-ketoadipate Pathway and the Biology of Selfidentity. Ann. Rev. Microbiol. 50, 553-590.
46. Hupert-Kocurek, K., Guzik, U. and Wojcieszynska, D. (2012). Characterization of catechol 2,3-dioxygenase from Planococcus sp. strain S5 induced by High Phenol Concentration. Acta Biochim. Pol. 59(3), 345-351.
47. Kargi, F. and Eker, S. (2004). Kinetics of 2,4-dichlorophenol Degradation by Pseudomonas putida CP1 in Batch Culture. Int. Biodet. Biodeg. 55, 25-28.
48. Karn, S.K., Chakrabarty, S.K. and Reddy, M.S. (2010). Pentachlorophenol Degradation by Pseudomonas stutzeri CL7 in the Secondary Sludge of Pulp and paper mill. J. Environ. Sci. 22(10), 1608-1612.
49. Khodadoust, A.P., Wanger, J.A., Suidan, M.T. and Brenner, R.C. (1997). Anaerobic Treatment of PCP in Fluidized-bed GAC Bioreactors. Water Res. 31, 1776-1786.
50. Kim, I.C. and Oriel, P.J. (1995). Characterization of the Bacillus stearothermophilus BR219 phenol hydroxylase gene. Appl. Environ. Microbiol. 61(4), 1252-1256.
51. Kobayashi, F., Maki, T. and Nakamura, Y. (2012). Biodegradation of Phenol in Seawater using Bacteria Isolated from the Intestinal contents of Marine Creatures. Int. Biodet. Biodeg. 69, 113-118.
52. Krastanov, A., Alexieva, Z. and Yemendzhiev, H. (2013). Microbial Degradation of Phenol and Phenolic Derivatives. Eng. Life Sci. 13, 76-87.
53. Krishnani, K.K., Parimala, V., Gupta, B.P., Azad, I.S., Meng, X. and Abraham, M. (2006). Bagasse-assisted Bioremediation of Ammonia from Shrimp Farm Wastewater. Water Environ. Res. 78, 938-950.
54. Kumar, A. and Kumar, S. (2005). Biodegradation Kinetics of Phenol and Catechol using Pseudomonas putida MTCC 1194. Biochem. Eng. J. 22, 151-159.
55. Kwon, K.H., Jung, K.Y. and Yeom, S.Y. (2009). Comparison between Entrapment methods for Phenol Removal and Operation of Bioreactor Packed with co-entrapped Activated Carbon and Pseudomonas Fluorescence KNU417. Bioprocess Biosyst. Eng. 32, 249-256.

56. Kwon, K.H. and Yeom, S.H. (2009). Optimal Microbial Adaptation Routes for the Rapid Degradation of High Concentration of Phenol. Bioprocess Biosyst. Eng. 32, 435-442.
57. Leonard, D. and Lindely, N.D. (1998). Growth of *Ralstonia eutropha* on Inhibitory Concentrations of Phenol-diminished Growth can be Attributed to Hydrophobic Perturbation of Phenol Hydroxylase Activity. Enz. Microbiol. Technol. 25, 271-277.
58. Li, H., Han, H., Du, M. and Wang, W. (2011). Removal of Phenols, Thiocyanate and Ammonium from Coal Gasification Wastewater using moving Bed Biofilm Reactor. Biores. Technol. 102(7), 4667-4673.
59. Li, H., Liu, T., Li, Z. and Deng, L. (2008). Low-cost Supports used to Immobilize Fungi and Reliable Technique for Removal Hexavalent Chromium in Wastewater. Biores. Technol. 99, 2234-2241.
60. Li, Y. and Wang, C. (2008). Phenol Biodegradation in Hybrid Hollow-fiber Membrane Bioreactors. World J. Biotechnol. 24, 1843-1849.
61. Limkhuansuwan, V. and Chaiprasert, P. (2010). Decolorization of Molasses Melanoidins and Palm Oil Mill Effluent Phenolic Compounds by Fermentative Lactic Acid Bacteria. J. Environ. Sci. 22(8), 1209-1217.
62. Liu, Y.J., Zhang, A.N. and Wang, X.C. (2009). Biodegradation of Phenol by using Free and Immobilized Cells of Acinetobacter sp. XA05 and Sphingomonas sp. FG03. Biochem. Eng. J. 44(2-3), 187-192.
63. Mamimin, C., Thongdumyu, P., Hniman, A., Prasertsan, P., Imai, T. and O-Thong, S. (2012). Simultaneous Thermophilic Hydrogen Production and Phenol Removal from Palm Oil Mill Effluent by Thermoanaerobacterium-rich Sludge. Int. J. Hydrogen Energy 37(20), 15598-15606.
64. Vennila, R. and Kannan, V. (2011). Bioremediation of Petroleum Refinery Effluent by Planococcus halophilus. African J. Biotechnol. 10(44), 8829-8833.
65. Wang, Y., Tian, Y., Han, B., Zhao, H.B., Bi, J.N. and Cai, B.L. (2007). Biodegradation of Phenol by Free and Immobilized Acinetobacter sp. strain PD12. J. Environ. Sci. 19, 222-225.
66. Wu, Z., Liu, Y., Liu, H., Xia, Y., Shen, W., Hong, Q., Li, S. and Yao, H. (2012). Characterization of the Nitrobenzene-degrading Strain Pseudomonas sp. a3 and use of its Immobilized Cells in the Treatment of mixed Aromatics Wastewater. World J. Microbiol. Biotechnol. 28(8), 2679-2687.
67. Zhao, G., Zhou, L., Li, Y., Liu, X., Ren, X. and Liu, X. (2009). Enhancement of Phenol Degradation using Immobilized Microorganisms and Organic modified Montmorillonite in a Two-phase Partitioning Bioreactor. J. Hazard. Mater. 169, 402-410.
68. Zhong, W., Wang, D. and Xu, X. (2012). Phenol Removal Efficiencies of Sewage Treatment Processes and Ecological Risks Associated with Phenols in Effluents. J. Hazard. Mater. (217- 218), 286-292.
69. Zoh, K. and Stenstrom, M.K. (2002). Application of a Membrane Bioreactor for Treating Explosives Process Wastewater. Water Res. 36(4), 1018-1024.

**Corresponding author: Murtaza Abid, Department of Botany, University of Lucknow, Lucknow, (U.P.,) India**
**Email: murtazaabid3@gmail.com**

# Index

**E**



**F**



**G**

❑❑❑❑❑

**PFS.** See Perfect Forward Secrecy

**PGP (Pretty Good Privacy).** A program used to encrypt and decrypt email over the Internet. It is also used to send an encrypted digital signature that lets the receiver verify the sender's identity and know that the message was not changed en route.

**PICS.** Platform for Internet Content Selection. A set of protocols developed by the World Wide Web consortium for communicating a rating for a Web, FTP or newsgroup server to an Internet client. PICS is intended to give users a method for categorizing, rating, and filtering Web and other Internet content. The protocols are extensions to both HTTP and HTML and allow users to customize selection criteria, or adopt, from a third party such as a Parent Teacher Association, established selection criteria or a list of sites to be screened out.

**ping (Packet Internet or Inter-Network Groper).** Basic Internet program that lets you verify that a particular IP address exists and can accept requests.

**pixel.** A single illuminated dot on a computer monitor.

**PKCS #11.** See Cryptoki.

**PKI Public Key Infrastructure.** A set of independent services to be developed by competing organizations that will support the use of Public Key in information security applications as well as in electronic commerce. The PKI will determine the policies for issuance of digital certificates, will issue and revoke certificates, and will save the information needed to subsequently validate the certificates. It will include certificate authorities organized both in hierarchies and in peer-to-peer networks.

**plain old telephone service (POTS).** The network connecting telephones; it provides a reliable data transmission bandwidth of about 56Kbps.

**platform.** A platform is an environment needed to run a piece of software. Thus the Windows Operating System serves as a platform for the Windows Office Suite. Further a browser would be considered a platform that a plug-in would need for it to function (thus Internet Explorer is a platform for Windows Media Player and Real Networks).

**plug-in.** Plug-in refers to additional software that is required to execute a transaction via a web browser. Thus if the webpage is designed to run with something that is not standard to the browser, the viewer needs to down load an additional plug-in. This may be used to run enhanced graphics (Flash), sound (Real Audio) or 3D (Cosmo Player), or other such rich media applications. Before designing to require a plug-in, it is important to note how much of your target audience has the additional plug-in, the likelihood of those not having the plug-in down loading it, and whether the design functions without the plug-in (i.e. does the additional feature(s) compliment or replace the information design of the site). As the web browser develops, the requirements of use of plug-ins will diminish, so this is a temporary situation. It is advised not to require the use of plug-ins on the homepage, especially if the information from the plug-in is required to meet the informational goals of the site.

**PNS.** See PPTP Network Server.

**Point-to-Point Tunneling Protocol (PPTP).** A call-control and management protocol that allows a PPTP Network Server to control access by dial-in circuit switched calls received by a PPTP Access Concentrator. It provides flow and congestion controlled encapsulation datagram service for carrying Point-to-Point Protocol packets. While PPTP does not provide encryption it can be used in conjunction with encryption to provide a Virtual Private Network over the Internet between an individual dialup user and a LAN or WAN.